Your Life in Your Hands

Your Life in Your Hands

Understanding, Preventing, and
Overcoming Breast Cancer

Jane A. Plant, Ph.D.

THOMAS DUNNE BOOKS ❦ NEW YORK
ST. MARTIN'S PRESS

THOMAS DUNNE BOOKS.
An imprint of St. Martin's Press.

www.stmartins.com

Design by Ellen Cipriano

The diagram of a breast on page 24 is reprinted from *Basic Anatomy and
Physiology* by H.G.Q. Rowett, by permission of John Murray (publishers) Ltd.
The painting on page 102, *Bathsheba with the Letter of David*, by
Rembrandt van Rijn (1606–1669), Louvre, Paris, France. Scala/Art Re-
source, New York.
The excerpt on page 239 from "Human Numbers, Environment,
Sustainability, and Health" by A. J. McMichael and J. W. Powles is re-
printed by permission from the *British Medical Journal*, October 1999.

LIBRARY OF CONGRESS CATALOGING-IN-PUBLICATION DATA
Plant, Jane A.
    Your life in your hands : understanding, preventing, and overcom-
ing breast cancer / Jane A. Plant.
        p.   cm.
Includes bibliographical references and index.
ISBN 0-312-27561-7
        1. Breast—Cancer—Popular works.   2. Breast—Cancer—Eti-
ology.   3. Breast—Cancer—Epidemiology.   4. Breast—Cancer—
Prevention.   5. Breast—Cancer—Diet therapy.   I. Title.

RC280.B8 P55 2001
616.99'449—dc21   00-047495

First published in Great Britain by Virgin Publishing Ltd.

First U.S. Edition: January 2001

10   9   8   7   6   5   4   3   2   1

For my children:
Mark,
Emma,
and Thomas

Author's Note

❦

The diagnosis and treatment of medical conditions are a responsibility shared by you and your medical advisers. All diets should begin with a medical checkup to make certain that no special health problems exist and to confirm that there are no medical reasons why you should not undertake a change of diet.

Contents

1. The Hat, The Boa Constrictor, and The Scientist   1

Why, as a natural scientist, I approach the problem of breast cancer differently than doctors and orthodox medical researchers. How my training and experience as an earth scientist helped me to cope with all the types of treatment a breast cancer patient is likely to undergo, including surgery, radiation therapy, and chemotherapy. Some of the mistakes I made and how to avoid them.

2. Cells Behaving Badly   52

What I wish I had been told when I was first diagnosed with breast cancer. Cancer explained clearly in unscary, everyday language based on information from recently published scientific papers.

3. The Third Strawberry   63

How I used my science, my knowledge, and my experience of working in China and Korea and with colleagues from these countries—as well as a large dollop of good luck—to identify what I believe to be the main factor promoting breast cancer.

4. Rich Woman's Disease   84

An explanation of the scientific evidence that links the consumption of dairy products to breast and prostate cancer. Why giving up dairy products can cut your risk of suffering from breast cancer, prostate cancer, and many other diseases.

5. The Plant Program—The Food Factors   114

The seven Food Factors that can help you cut your risk of suffering from breast or prostate cancer.

6. The Plant Program—The Lifestyle Factors   198

The five Lifestyle Factors that can help you cut your risk of breast or prostate cancer. These range from reducing stress to reducing your exposure to man-made chemicals.

7. Reflections from West to East   232

Why "the system" has failed to protect us from, or even inform us of, the many avoidable risk factors implicated in breast and prostate cancer. Ten Golden Guidelines to follow to reduce risk—both individual and societal. Why women's lives really are in their own hands.

Acknowledgments

❧

Jane A. Plant acknowledges the help and support of family, friends, and colleagues at the British Geological Survey, especially the director, Dr. David Falvey. I am particularly grateful to Ruth Cavin for her excellent work in producing the U.S. edition of this book. The original manuscript was typed by Kathe Fairhurst.

Welcome

❧

This book has come about as a result of many hundreds of conversations I have had with women who want answers.

Breast cancer is a puzzling, and frightening, subject. As someone who has suffered five times from progressively more advanced breast cancer, which eventually spread to my lymph system before it was finally defeated, I know from firsthand experience just how terrifying it can be. But although breast cancer is a subject that frightens many women, this is *not* a frightening book. Quite the opposite, in fact: it is empowering and optimistic. It is a story of hope.

Over the past century, Western women have achieved extraordinary progress in a great many areas. We now have the power to vote for our governance and the methods to plan our families and to ensure that a high proportion of our children survive, and we can be educated alongside men in any subject we choose. Despite all these impressive and valuable gains, today's "epidemic" of breast cancer now jeopardizes our well-being, assaults the very symbols of our femininity and motherhood, and indeed menaces our lives as few other threats do.

The facts are stark and shocking. For adult women (aged between 25 and 75) the leading cause of death is cancer[1]: and the type of cancer that kills most women is breast cancer.[2] Out of about every ten women you know, one of them (I hope, not you) is likely to contract breast cancer.[3] These dry statistics actually understate the severity of the situation because breast cancer affects the lives of far more people than that: when you include all the spouses, sons, daughters, mothers, fathers, friends, colleagues, and loved ones whose lives are blighted by this disease, then you begin to realize just what a modern-day scourge we are dealing with. Almost no one in the Western world can consider themselves immune from its impact. Indeed, our increasing affluence appears to make matters worse. Most diseases affect the poorer rather than the wealthier, more educated members of society, but breast and prostate cancer are different. They mainly affect the higher socioeconomic groups.[4] Indeed, the slang name for breast cancer in China translates as "Rich Woman's Disease" as it mainly attacks women who follow a Western middle-class lifestyle.

For too long women have unquestioningly accepted that a proportion of us will be affected by breast cancer. We have been persuaded to be too passive about prevention, accepting the idea that there is little or nothing we can do ourselves to prevent a disease that, quite literally, decimates the female population. And the overwhelming majority of our medical, scientific, political, and financial efforts are directed toward detecting and treating, rather than preventing, this awful disease.

The message you'll read in these pages is very different.

I believe that all women have the right to the best available information so that they can make informed decisions for themselves. My aim in this book is to set before you, clearly and plainly, vital information that can help you drastically cut your risk of contracting—and dying from—breast cancer. One of the frustrations for most women is not knowing how to help themselves. We know that if we smoke we increase our risk of lung cancer and if we sunbathe too much we increase our risk of skin cancer, so we can choose whether to take these risks. But in the case of breast cancer, we are too often made to feel helpless because we are rarely told about anything we can do to protect ourselves. Although we are told of many risk factors for breast cancer, they do not translate into anything we can actually do. This makes us feel powerless.

For the first time, this book makes available to all women a compelling body of new evidence that points to the underlying causes of breast cancer. It is my hope that women will use this information to prevent or treat this disease in themselves or those close to them. There is much useful information gleaned from my own personal experience on the very practical aspects of dealing with the disease, including diagnosis and treatment. In addition, I have observed in my research that much of the data and information about prostate cancer leads to conclusions similar to those regarding the cause and treatment of breast cancer. Anticipating the care that the women who read this will extend to the men in their lives, I have included much about prostate cancer. You will also find suggestions on how by changing values and behavior patterns, with the aim of improving the environment, we can reduce our exposure as a society to some of the factors that may contribute to these diseases.

This book chronicles, in part, my journey through five progressively worse episodes of breast cancer and describes how I used my training as a scientist to cope with both the disease and the treatments I was given for it. That scientific training had taught me to observe and record everything, to root out every fragment of information, to sift the relevant from the irrelevant, the rational from the irrational, and to keep asking those two key questions that are at the very heart of science: why and how? This book contains what I believe to be the answers to those two questions regarding breast cancer.

If this book had been around even two years before my first diagnosis of breast cancer, I am sure that I would never have had the disease. I hope very much that you can put the information it contains to the best possible use in your own life.

Before you begin, it might help if I give you a few tips on how to use the book. The first chapter is about my knowledge and experience as a scientist and as a breast cancer sufferer.

Chapters 2 and 4 provide scientific information aimed especially at health professionals wishing to help their patients. The information is mainly from peer-reviewed gold standard scientific literature translated into simple, straightforward English. Many women who are not scientists but who want to know the basis for my approach have enjoyed reading the information and found it helpful.

If, however, you have active cancer and just want to grasp the essentials as quickly as possible, you may wish to begin at Chapter 3 and then read Chapters 5 and 6.

The last chapter is about the politics of it all, just to remind everyone that some scientific messages are there to confuse. (There is now mounting information about how the tobacco industry funded research to confuse people about the health effects of smoking tobacco.) I should like to reassure everyone that I wrote the book on my own time with no funding or influence from any vested interest group, and did my best to ensure that the science I used was, to the best of my knowledge, objective, authoritative, and as free as possible from commercial or political influences.

Your Life in Your Hands

1.

The Hat,
The Boa Constrictor,
and The Scientist

In this chapter I explain to you why, as a natural scientist, I approach the problem of breast cancer differently than doctors and orthodox medical researchers. I then go on to explain how I used my training and experience to cope with all the orthodox types of treatment a breast cancer patient is likely to undergo, including surgery, radiation therapy, and chemotherapy. I explain the treatments clearly and simply and give lots of practical tips to help you cope: for example, how to avoid or minimize hair loss during chemotherapy. In this chapter I have tried to make you feel as if you have a good and caring friend guiding you toward the light at the end of the tunnel.

Scientists can often seem to be rather strange people.

The truth is, scientists are different—we're trained to be. Let me explain what I mean by using the story I tell when I first lecture to new students at one of the universities I visit. It comes from a wonderful children's story you may already be familiar with: *The Little Prince* by Antoine de Saint-Exupéry. In this magical book the little prince draws a

I pondered deeply, then, over the adventures of the jungle. And after some work with a coloured pencil I succeeded in making my first drawing. My drawing Number One. It looked like this:

picture of a boa constrictor digesting an elephant. But when he shows his masterpiece to grown-ups and asks them whether they are frightened by the picture, they ask why they should be frightened by a picture of a hat. It is the ability to see that the hat is a boa constrictor digesting an elephant that distinguishes the best scientists.

Let me give you a well-known example to show you what I mean. What sort of person sees an apple fall from a tree, wonders what force is drawing it down toward the earth—and then goes on to develop the whole concept of gravity?

Here's another example. What sort of person leaves a plate of glass coated with photographic emulsion next to a piece of granite in a drawer and, when he notices that the emulsion appears to have been damaged by "emanations" coming from the granite, does not simply curse and throw it away but instead deduces that previously unknown particles and rays have been emitted from the rock—and discovers radioactivity?

And one more. What sort of person attempts to culture bacteria in a petri dish, finds the experiment has gone "moldy," yet does not simply throw it away but instead looks carefully, observes that something in the fungus has killed the bacteria, and discovers penicillin—thereby establishing the basis for the development of modern antibiotics?

All three people—Sir Isaac Newton, Henri Bequerel, and Sir Alexander Fleming—saw things a little bit differently. It is this ability to see a familiar situation from a different viewpoint or angle that probably makes scientists seem rather odd to other people. But sometimes it results in a major leap forward in our understanding of the natural world.

Thinking like a creative scientist is more a state of mind than anything to do with training or education (although increasingly, we need to know and understand more and more facts before we can contribute new ideas).

This book sees things a little bit differently. For many decades, women have lived in the shadow of a devastating disease that continues to kill a high proportion of sufferers and that is associated in many women's minds with treatments involving invasive surgery, irradiation, or chemicals with frightening side effects. The disease is, of course, breast cancer. The only hope we are given is that with enough expenditure on research, we might one day find a truly effective treatment. Sadly, that day has been a very long time coming.

In these pages I want to take you on a journey. Partly it is the story of my own learning experiences with breast cancer, which I have suffered from five times and eventually conquered. But mainly it is the story of a new and rather different way of seeing, understanding, and treating this disease.

It is my hope that this book will serve two purposes. First, I want it to be directly useful to you, the reader. The straightforward advice and simple lifestyle suggestions it contains will be of practical benefit to *every woman* in significantly reducing the risk of developing breast cancer. If you happen to be that one woman in ten who has developed breast cancer, then you will also find much additional information here, which will give you a better chance of survival overall and help you to cope with rigorous treatment methods.

Second, it is vitally important that this book ignite a debate within the scientific and medical communities. Science is, at heart, an adversarial process. Progress is made by vigorous cross-questioning of your own and others' work. This book puts forward a new perspective on breast and prostate cancer and backs it up with compelling evidence from the scientific literature. The inescapable conclusion is that relatively small augmentations to the orthodox medical therapies currently being used in clinics and hospitals would result in major improvements in patient survival. For example, providing breast cancer patients with sound dietary advice, as is common in the case of heart disease or diabetes, could greatly increase survival rates. So much suffering could be prevented, and so many lives could be saved, that the evidence must be heard—and acted upon—with the very greatest urgency.

HOW MY STORY BEGAN

I didn't choose to study breast cancer—it chose me.

I first stumbled into science because I was an instinctive feminist. The boys at my local grammar school could choose among Latin, art, and physics as options, while at the girls' school we could choose from only Latin, art, and cookery. Although Latin was my best subject, I did not like it and resented the time spent on something that, as a teenager, I could see little point in. So I led a campaign for the girls to be offered the same choices as the boys and, for my efforts, became hoist with my own petard when I was obliged to study physics just as the boys did. Without quite realizing it, I had started on the road to becoming a scientist.

At school I occasionally regretted what I had done, but at university I literally fell in love with the scientific subject I had chosen to do— geochemistry. I was the only woman to pursue the subject in the final year; however, I was so dedicated and such a perfectionist that I had some problems. For example, after my final year examinations I ran away because I believed I had failed my exams. In fact, when my professor finally tracked me down it was to tell me that I had gained a first class honors degree.

After leaving university I married a young doctor who subsequently trained as an army psychiatrist, and had a son, named Mark. Our marriage failed and, in a protracted and painful custody battle, I lost my son to my ex-husband and his new wife, a psychologist. This has been a source of intense and chronic stress for the last thirty years of my life. Four years after we separated, I married my present husband, Peter, who, like me, is an earth scientist. We have two children, Emma, now twenty-five, and Tom, now eighteen. You will read about them later.

I was lucky to be employed by the British Geological Survey (BGS) as only the second woman scientist in its history. (Women had previously been employed only in a technical capacity.) I am now the Chief Scientist of the organization, and I hope my position is helping to encourage other women to progress in what in the past has been a very male-dominated subject.

Geochemistry is about the chemistry of the earth. My specialty is in

understanding the chemistry of the surface of the earth, especially concentrations of chemicals where these occur either as natural concentrations
in ore deposits or as a result of man's activity; for example, where there
are landfill sites or contaminated land. I have frequently worked with
biochemists, veterinarians, epidemiologists, and medical geographers looking at the impact of chemicals in the environment on the health of humans, animals, and crops. Early in my career, between 1975 and 1977, I
served on a Royal Society committee concerned with geochemistry and
health.[1] Since that time, my team of scientists at the British Geological
Survey has been concerned with a wide range of human health problems
related to the environment. Some of the methods we have developed allow
us to make highly reproducible high-resolution maps showing the distribution of chemicals over the surface of the earth. We are able to look on
our computer screens at the distribution of, say, arsenic and uranium (as
potentially toxic elements) or zinc or iron (trace elements essential to
animal and human health) in the same way people can look at Earth's
physiography—using remotely sensed photographs from space.[2] Almost
from the beginning, these images, although intended for geologists, created a lot of interest among veterinarians, who found them helpful in
diagnosing environmental and nutritional animal diseases in Britain. It
was by working with them that I first began to learn of some of the
amazing connections between geochemistry and biochemistry. I also
learned, when I was ill, that veterinary rather than medical literature provided the most fundamental answers based on biochemistry. Eventually I
established a team that is regarded as the best in the world in tackling
health problems related to anomalous levels of trace elements in the
environment—for example, diseases caused by high levels of arsenic or
fluoride or by deficiencies in iodine, selenium, cobalt, or zinc in soils and/
or water supplies. This is a particular problem in many developing countries.

Very recent work that the BGS team has conducted, which has received wide publicity, deals with the problem of arsenic contamination in
water from wells in Bangladesh. There the levels of arsenic in water can
be so high that many people develop skin lesions—their skin becomes
black and thickened—that in a significant proportion of sufferers become
cancerous.

What I had learned as a result of this type of environmental detective work time and time again was that until you identified the *fundamental cause* of such problems, there was little or nothing that could be done to help the affected individuals. And until you've found the cause (whether it's of breast cancer or any other disease) and effectively neutralized it, you can never, ever claim to have "solved" the problem.

Until 1987 I had no interest in cancer because, like most people, I never imagined that it could happen to me. I had never smoked or sunbathed, rarely drank alcohol, and ate what most experts would consider to be a healthy diet. I even checked to make sure that the cosmetics I used contained no harmful chemicals. My lifestyle was hectic, certainly (it still is!), but no more stressful than many other women's.

Then, one Friday evening in September of that year, my life changed forever.

I was in northern Canada examining gold deposits before attending a major scientific conference in Toronto. I was working on a project aimed at understanding how gold, which is the rarest element on earth, could become concentrated by factors of up to about 10,000 times by natural geologic processes to form minable gold deposits. I was feeling pleased because I had begun to see clues that would lead to new theories and models, which subsequently I published in peer-reviewed papers (see p. 15) and in a textbook I wrote over the next few years. It had been a grueling day working down in the gold mine. It was hot, sweaty, dirty work, not to mention noisy and dusty, and I couldn't wait to get back to my hotel and the luxury of soap, hot water, and fresh towels.

Finally back in my room, I dried myself and returned to my bedroom to search for a bra. As I was walking around topless hunting for my underwear, I suddenly saw in the low-angle, late-afternoon sunlight a lump about the size of a large pea just under the skin of my left breast. I felt it and was immediately overwhelmed with fear and panic; my mouth went dry and I felt sick. I knew without a doubt that I had breast cancer. Over the next week or so, I was to become very familiar with the feel of the cancer. I was surprised by how hard it felt—like a compressed rubber ball surrounding one of the ducts in my left breast. I was angry with myself for not having examined my breasts before, but somehow I had never thought the advice applied to me. I was only 42—surely too young to get cancer? My family and loved ones, my developing career, the many happy and productive years I had always imagined to be ahead of me . . . In one heart-stopping moment, everything came crashing to a very full stop.

After the initial shock had subsided somewhat, I tried to think what to do. My husband was working in Jamaica and I had no contact telephone number (this is common among geologists), and my children were both staying with their grandmother. In any case, I saw no point in upsetting them. The first thing I did was to telephone one of my oldest and dearest friends. Dr. John Camac had been my doctor throughout my childhood and was still my mother's doctor. Despite the fact that it must have been about midnight in Britain, he was wonderful to me. He guided me through a careful self-examination. He knew me well enough not to give me false reassurances and we agreed that the lump that I had found probably was cancer but that it appeared to be very localized and could probably be treated by lumpectomy on my return to Britain. With his advice and the help of a friend in Canada, I decided to stay for the conference until I had honored my commitments, but also to go to the famous Princess Margaret Hospital in Toronto for an examination and diagnosis.

I thus spent the next week alternately being a professional scientist chairing sessions or giving lectures in front of an audience of about 800 people; attending a specialist breast clinic for examinations and biopsies, finally to be given the diagnosis of cancer; and sitting alone or with friends feeling like a terrified 5-year-old worrying about what the future held. Most people have some attractive feature—for example, long legs, beautiful hair or eyes, and so on. In my case, it had been my boobs. I had a small waist and shapely breasts. Before I was married, my surname was Lunn and this led to two of my teenage nicknames—busty Lunn or lusty bun! The thought of losing one of my breasts terrified me. Would it mean that people would treat me as an object of pity? Would my colleagues joke about me?

By the time I returned to London, my local doctor had already managed to get me an appointment with the breast cancer clinic in a leading London teaching hospital, the Charing Cross Hospital. I shall never forget the scene that greeted me on my first visit. The waiting room was full to bursting with strained-looking women and their supporters; the atmosphere was thick with fear and anxiety; there was no conversation, and mostly we avoided even making eye contact with each other. Even then,

I noted that most of the women appeared well groomed but were of different ages, different shapes and builds, and with different breast sizes. There were two black women, one woman of Indian appearance, one woman of Middle Eastern appearance, but no Eastern women. Looking back I realize that I was already searching for clues about the cause of breast cancer by looking for common factors among the women affected. Of course, if it were that easy someone would have identified the factors long ago, but it was impossible for me to suppress my instincts as a scientist. Seeing those scared faces—and knowing how scared I felt, too— was the first time I fully understood what a common disease breast cancer is, and how dreadful and widespread is the damage it causes to women and their families and friends.

Over the months and years that followed my first visit to that clinic, I made it my business to learn as much as I could about this devastating disease. In times of great personal crisis, people usually fall back on the fundamental things they know best and trust most. For some, it may be their religious faith. For others, it could be close friends and loved ones. In my case, when disaster struck, I fell back on what I trusted most: my scientific training.

And that's what saved my life.

HOW SCIENCE SERVES US— AND WHY IT SOMETIMES DOESN'T

A good scientist will see things a little bit differently from most people. As a science "insider," I'd like to tell you something about the way science works, which will help you make sense of the differing approaches that scientists have adopted toward breast cancer.

When I lecture to my students, I like to ask them to visualize science as a mighty oak tree—a tree of knowledge, if you like. Start deep down under the earth, at the very tips of the ever-probing roots. This is where lots of discoveries are constantly being made and new facts found. Then some of these are brought together to form larger roots, and finally, the whole knowledge can be assembled to give a total or holistic trunk to the tree. This last function—the assembling of disparate bits of information to give a new insight or theory or sometimes a major breakthrough—has often been achieved by one individual with a grasp of many or all of the different aspects of a problem, who has the good fortune to be in the right place at the right time to make all the necessary connections. Finally, this newly acquired knowledge flows to the branches and leaves, as the information is communicated to the world at large—where it may be used for good or ill.

This is, of course, a simplification of a complex and dynamic subject, but it is a useful way of understanding how science has always functioned to deliver the fruits of its labors to society. In recent years, however, things have changed significantly, and not for the better. Today, the overwhelming trend is to devote maximum attention and resources (money, people, equipment, and facilities) to scientists working at the root tips, often using very expensive, high-technology methods. Sometimes this approach is called "bottom-up" science (as opposed to "top-down"). The great natural scientist James E. Lovelock lucidly explains the problem in his book *Gaia: The Practical Science of Planetary Medicine:* "To understand the physiology of the earth requires a 'top-down' view of the earth as a whole system. We need science, but it must grow from the top down as well as the bottom up!"

Science that exclusively and narrowly focuses on the extreme root tips at the expense of everything else can be bad science. My friend Professor John Dewey FRS, of Oxford University, made this point recently in a thoughtful and thought-provoking article in the science journal *Geoscientist* (John is a modern scientific hero, being one of the pioneers of plate tectonic theory, which explains how the earth's surface has evolved over time). He wrote:

In our ambitious scramble for funds and recognition, we have forgotten the traditional values of scholarship, the seamless integration of research and teaching to generate knowledge and science. Scholarship includes intense library research and reading literature more than five years old.[3]

There is a word to describe what has happened to many branches of science in recent decades, which is increasingly used pejoratively: reductionism.

The current emphasis on high-technology reductionist science means, to put it candidly, that we are spending more and more to learn more and more about less and less. As far as cancer research is concerned, it means that we are studying ever smaller parts of the total process involved in the development of the disease, such as some aspect of cell biology or molecular chemistry—in some cases just one gene, or the protein it encodes for. But this increasing specialization and compartmentalization of cancer research, each subdivision with its own jargon (which other researchers may not understand), simply isn't producing the results that society is entitled to.

There's another problem caused by the emphasis on reductionist science, too. Its all-pervading influence has made any other type of scientific endeavor more difficult to pursue. In particular, I'm talking about the sort of science that takes place further up the tree trunk—the sort of science that involves analyzing, synthesizing, or reviewing the work of others. This is now highly unfashionable. It is thought not to be creative and not to provide the original cutting-edge ideas that "bottom-up" science produces. Hence there are few prizes or distinctions for scientists carrying out such tasks, and it is difficult to find sources of funding for this type of work.

The implied aim of reductionist science, in the case of cancer research, is to find the single "magic bullet," that one missing piece of the jigsaw, the ultimate answer, the Holy Grail.

But what if it doesn't exist?

In the meantime, we are left with surgery, radiation therapy, and chemotherapy—albeit improved and refined—as the main front-line treatments against breast cancer, as they have been since the 1950s, together with hormone-based methods such as the drug tamoxifen. True, there have been small, incremental improvements, but little that is having much impact on the incidence of breast cancer or affecting the long-term survival of many sufferers (see Fig. 1, p. 74).

A reductionist approach to breast cancer research also, sooner or later, runs into the law of diminishing returns, whereby we have to spend more and more economic resources in order to achieve less and less.

The high-technology approach to developing drugs for cancer is leading to many new drugs that are extremely expensive—which are then strongly marketed, often directly to patients via the World Wide Web— although they may prolong life for only a few weeks or months. Hence there are increasingly highly charged emotional debates between individual patients and their families, who understandably wish to have the latest treatment, and health authorities and organizations that find it difficult to justify the large aggregated bills for groups of patients receiving marginal benefit. Is this approach really helpful to breast cancer sufferers except in the very short term?

The modern era in cancer research really began in America when President Richard Nixon proclaimed "war" on cancer in his State of the Union address in 1971. And right from the beginning, it was dominated by reductionist scientific thinking, with its requirement for large-scale funding, extracted with the beguiling promise of a cure "just round the corner." "Many people anticipated swift victory," recounts the newsmagazine *U.S. News & World Report*, with the taming of the dread disease likened to a moon landing. Even as recently as 1984, the National Cancer Institute's director predicted that cancer deaths could be halved by the year 2000 in America.

Such optimism was, of course, unjustified. Despite massive expenditure—$2 billion in the United States in 1996 alone—by 1992 the cancer death rate had risen by more than 6 percent.[4] Adopting the battlefield metaphor so beloved of cancer scientists, some critics have called Nixon's war on cancer a "medical Vietnam."

Certainly, there have been some significant medical success stories. For example, childhood cancers, particularly some leukemias, can now be treated and cured quite effectively: between 75 and 80 percent of children diagnosed with acute lymphocytic leukemia can now be cured. But these bright spots are too few and far between.

So what, you may be wondering, is the alternative to relying so heavily on reductionist science? And is it any more effective in delivering tangible benefits to ordinary people?

Most doctors would agree that the greatest contribution to all mankind in overcoming infectious diseases came not from the use of antibiotics but from improvements in public health: a clean water supply, improved sanitation, better nutrition, and proper housing. These improvements came about as we gradually increased our understanding of why and how infectious diseases were transmitted. An early example of this type of work was carried out by Dr. John Snow, who showed the value of studying the pattern of occurrence of disease. He made the famous dot map that showed the location of deaths from the epidemic of cholera that occurred in central London in September 1854. Deaths were marked by dots, and the area's eleven water pumps were located by crosses. Examining the scatter over the surface of the map, Snow observed that cholera occurred almost entirely among those who lived near (and drank from) the Broad Street water pump. He had the handle of the contaminated pump removed, ending the neighborhood epidemic, which had taken more than 500 lives. This "scientific detective work" is called epidemiology—literally the study of epidemics—and it has been used successfully many times to identify the cause of disease and, through public health medicine, to correct the things society was doing wrong.

In the case of cancer, Professor Sir Richard Doll's epidemiological study of lung cancer in the 1950s was one of the most significant advances in understanding cancer in this century. Sir Richard Doll demonstrated beyond any shadow of a doubt the relationship between lung cancer and smoking tobacco. Lung cancer was shown not to be a curse visited on us by a wrathful God, nor to occur because of bad or faulty genes, but rather to be caused by something human beings were doing to themselves. For the first time we had a modern rationale and scientific understanding of the cause of a common type of cancer. Following Doll's work, we can now choose whether to smoke or not in the knowledge that by doing so we shall significantly increase our risk of getting lung cancer. Moreover, identifying the cause of lung cancer has caused people in the United Kingdom to quit smoking, halving the death rate from lung cancer there.[5] Since that time, rational explanations have been found for many other types of cancers. For example, mesothelioma—a type of chest wall cancer—is now known to be caused by exposure to asbestos dust, skin cancer to be caused by exposure to ultraviolet light or arsenic poisoning, and cervical cancer to be caused by infection with the sexually transmitted human papilloma (wart) virus, to give but a few examples.

All this background information suddenly becomes much more than an academic discussion when you've just had a diagnosis of breast cancer.

The first thing I did after my initial diagnosis was to fill out a questionnaire, which established that I was at low risk of contracting breast cancer! According to the Breast Cancer Society of Canada and Statistics Canada, some of the main risk factors are:

+ Family history of breast cancer, especially in mothers, daughters, and sisters, as well as relatives such as aunts, cousins, and grand-mothers. There is a six-times-greater risk if a mother or sister had breast cancer prior to menopause and up to ten-times-greater risk if the cancer was in both breasts for a mother or sister.
+ A *slightly* higher risk for women who have never carried a full-term pregnancy or whose first pregnancy was after age 30.
+ A higher risk with the early onset of menstruation or late onset of menopause.

Other suggested risk factors include prolonged use of the contraceptive pill before the first child, a history of benign breast lumps, the use of hormone replacement therapy (HRT), a high consumption of alcohol, obesity, and increased age.

In fact, most of these risk factors translate into indicators of a Western middle-class lifestyle and may not mean very much. Let me explain. Before Professor Doll's work, which showed that lung cancer was associated with tobacco smoking, a set of risk factors similar to those quoted for breast cancer could have been developed for lung cancer. In the 1950s, before Professor Doll reported his findings, these would probably have included being male (at the time few women smoked), being working class, consuming alcohol, increasing age, coming from a family where others had had lung cancer (smokers tend to have parents who smoke), and so on. None of the risk factors *caused* lung cancer—they were simply features of the population who smoked. I believe that the situation with breast cancer risk factors is the same: they are *descriptions* of the population that contracts breast cancer.

Many doctors tend to see noncommunicable diseases, especially breast and prostate cancer, as simply an inevitable result of aging. For example, a recent article in the *British Medical Journal* spoke of "the growing burden of non-communicable disease—in both developed and developing countries—as a consequence of population ageing. Cardiovascular disease, cancer, neuropsychiatric conditions, and injury are fast becoming the leading causes of disability and premature death in most regions."[6] There is no mention in

the article of the influence of Western diet and lifestyle or other possible underlying causes of noncommunicable diseases. According to this line of reasoning, age is a primary cause of cancer. I, for one, don't believe it.

In the period that followed my initial diagnosis, a grim sort of race
ensued. As I suffered five times from progressively more advanced breast
cancer, which eventually spread to my lymph system, I was simultaneously
searching for greater scientific understanding of my disease, what might
have caused it, and what might effectively make it disappear.

At the start I was very, very frightened. I kept questioning the basis
of the therapy I was prescribed, investigating the data on outcomes myself,
and as far as I could, evaluating all possible alternative therapies and
theories. None of this made life easy for the cancer specialists treating me,
but it made all the difference in the world to me. I felt less of a victim,
and looking back I realize that this approach saved my life.

Sometimes I became very confused indeed. At the time there were
seriously conflicting views among medical professionals on the value of
mastectomy versus lumpectomy, just as recently there has been a major
controversy about the value of expenditure on mammography versus improving chemotherapy. Then there is the undeclared state of war that
seems to exist between orthodox and complementary (alternative) medicine about what to do for the best, so that you can quickly and easily
become entirely bewildered.

What was I to do? The only course of action that made any sense to
me and gave me any feeling of security was to fall back on my scientific
training.

Customarily, scientists approach a new problem in five stages:

1. **Gather existing information.** Review previous facts and theories
   as objectively and impartially but as critically as possible.
2. **Produce new information.** This is collected by experiment or observations, without emotional involvement. In some cases new
   ideas are produced by analysis and synthesis of information produced by other scientists. To be a good scientist you must be
   prepared to admit you are wrong: arriving at the truth is what is
   important, not personal prestige. If you raise a question, even if
   you arrive at the wrong answer, you will be respected if you work
   with honesty and openness. At the beginning of my science career,

I learned a saying that has always stayed with me and guided my work: "The person who asks the questions solves the problem."

3. **Evaluate.** Evaluate the new results in relation to existing theories, and identify new insights or ideas.

4. **Propose a new hypothesis.** Speculation must be identified as such and clearly separated from facts.

5. **Test the hypothesis.** If the hypothesis works, submit it for further testing and validation until you have a new theory. If it doesn't work, begin again.

In a recently published paper, Dr. D. E. Packham of the University of Bath listed the characteristic values to which scientists have traditionally aspired:[7]

+ Honest experimentation
+ Meticulous respect for evidence
+ Candid admission of mistakes or error
+ Pursuit of truth
+ Moral and intellectual independence of all political authority and economic power
+ Openness to the public scrutiny of research by one's peers. (You will see that throughout the book I use the term *peer reviewed* to indicate science published after it has been critically reviewed by other scientists. This type of information is distinguished from newspaper reports and other sources of information.)

This logical and ethical framework has been successfully used by scientists (whether they realized it or not) for centuries. And it is precisely how I began to approach the challenge of my own breast cancer.

What I discovered in the months and years that followed the diagnosis of my breast cancer is the subject of the rest of this book. There is indeed a great wealth of accumulated research—some of which goes back many decades—on the factors involved in breast and prostate cancer. As you read the chapters that follow, I am sure you will be just as astonished as I was initially to learn precisely how much has been discovered already but has not filtered through to the public. While it is true that some of the risk factors for breast cancer—such as increasing age, early age of onset of menstruation, late age of onset of menopause, and family history of breast cancer—are completely outside our control, there are many other risk factors that we can control—easily. These controllable risk factors readily translate into simple changes that we can all make in our day-to-day lives to help prevent or treat breast cancer.

My message is: Even advanced breast cancer can be overcome.

I know, because I've done it.

HOW MY STORY CONTINUED

What follows is what happened to me after that first fateful diagnosis: what I did wrong, what I did right, and what I'd do differently if I knew then what I know today. I shall also explain the reasoning and rationale for current cancer therapy and describe exactly how it felt to be a cancer patient.

One of the first questions I asked, one that many women with experience of breast cancer will understand, is "Why me? Why has this awful thing happened to me?" Eventually I found the answer to this question, and it was very disquieting because it brought home to me the high risk I had been running, despite what I'd thought was a healthy lifestyle. However, as I was to learn, a Western woman's lifestyle increases her risk of developing breast cancer, the risk increasing more and more every year.

Throughout the West, breast cancer is the most commonly occurring cancer affecting women.[8] In the United States, breast cancer is second only to lung cancer as a cause of cancer deaths among women. In the European Union, it is the commonest cancer affecting women, and three times more women will be affected by breast cancer than by the second-in-line killer, bowel cancer. Breast cancer is relatively rare in women under age 25, and more than four out of five women affected are older than 50. Breast cancer remains the leading cause of cancer death in women between the ages of 40 and 55 in many Western countries. A small number of men—a few hundred a year—also develop breast cancer.

Looked at another way, in the West the risk of any woman developing breast cancer during her lifetime varies from about one in eight in parts of the United States, to about one in twenty in parts of southern Europe.

For women in the United Kingdom, the risk is about one in twelve. Disturbingly, the risk has increased quite considerably in recent decades. For example, breast cancer attacked one woman in twenty in the United States in 1960, but by 1991 the rate was one in nine (and it is even higher there now).[9] Between 1979 and 1987 the rates in the United Kingdom increased at approximately 2 percent per annum, but between 1988 and 1992 the annual rate of increase rose to nearly 4.5 percent.[10]

So I should not have been so surprised to be one of those affected. The odds were high. However, what struck me very forcibly when I first became aware of these figures was the contrast between the comparatively high risk Western women run of contracting breast cancer and the much lower risk of women living in the East (see Chapter 3). This was my first suspicion that there might be a *cause* for breast cancer, just as there is a specific cause for the high risk of lung cancer that smokers run. In the following chapters, I will tell you what I think that is, but first, let us go along the orthodox path of treatment that most breast cancer sufferers will follow to a greater or lesser extent, depending on the type of cancer they are suffering from and the stage it has reached.

HOLDING YOUR GROUND

The typical route through cancer treatment is surgery, radiation therapy, and chemotherapy. My therapy was typical: radical mastectomy, three further operations, thirty-five radiation therapy treatments, five irradiations of my ovaries to induce menopause and eliminate my own estrogen, and twelve chemotherapy treatments. This all sounds like a barrage of therapies; and indeed, some alternative therapists use the analogy of breast cancer treatment as a battle between the disease and the treatments—with the patient as the battlefield. Although this analogy is not popular with cancer charities or doctors, one of the things you must realize from the outset is the heavy toll that surgery, anesthesia, radiation therapy, and chemotherapy will take on your body. Many people have to take breaks or give up treatments, especially chemotherapy courses, because they become too ill—for example, their blood cell counts fall to too low a level. The treatments can be particularly difficult for men with the disease if the only clinics available to them are for women. To cope with treatment you need to be equipped physically, emotionally, and practically. Dietary and other methods to keep my body as well nourished as possible helped me cope physically. Using my scientific knowledge I developed other coping strategies to ensure that radioactive substances (used for diagnosis) or chemotherapeutic substances (used for treatment) were removed from my body as soon as possible after they had done their job. I outline these coping strategies in a "tips" section at the end of this chapter. I have found that other breast cancer sufferers find such tips very helpful.

A VICTIM NO MORE

Cancer patients often feel as if the disease is their fault—either a genetic defect, something to do with "blocked emotions" (research shows that there's no such thing as a "cancer personality"—see Chapter 6), or the result of some other personal failing. This isn't true. Additionally, conventional cancer therapy can "process" patients to the extent that they no longer understand what is really being done to them. A cancer patient is a vulnerable person, and the relentless procedures may induce a feeling of loss of control. But it is vitally important to retain control and develop a constructive working partnership with your doctor. Let me show you how I stopped being a victim, refused to hand over control to my doctors, and set out to discover more about the "big C" force that appeared to be driving me relentlessly toward death.

In the case of breast cancer it is important to understand the different roles of research scientists, including medical researchers, and clinical doctors. Doctors are professional human biologists who have taken an oath—the Hippocratic oath—which requires that they follow a strict code of ethical and professional behavior. They tend to use only orthodox procedures that have been established by clinical trials, usually based on pure chemical substances or standardized technical procedures and validated by well-controlled, statistically based experiments using cell cultures or laboratory animals and, finally, patients. The growing threat of litigation against medical practitioners is making it more and more difficult for them to depart from orthodox medicine (although a recent series of articles about alternative medicine in the *British Medical Journal* shows the increasing acceptance of some of these methods by a profession that is necessarily conservative). Ideas such as using diet to treat illness go back to the Hippocratic School of Medicine that originated in Greece in about 400 B.C. Hippocrates scorned the belief that disease is caused by magical or supernatural forces and said that everything had a rational origin. He suggested that the causes of disease lay in air, water, and food and noted the body's ability to heal itself given the right conditions related to these natural factors. Indeed, there is an argument that modern Western medicine's departure from these traditional roots began with the use of surgery during the American Civil War. Natural substances have been used in Chinese medicine for more than 3,000 years. As the World Health Organization has pointed out, most of the people on earth still rely on herbal treatments.

Like most groups of professionals, doctors range in their ability from excellent to poor. My experience with medical doctors encompasses both and is probably typical. I was fortunate in some ways because right from the beginning I was not in awe of them as many patients are. Even before I embarked on a career in science, I had developed something of a questioning approach toward medical custom and convention, which probably stemmed from my father's treatment at the hands of psychiatrists. He was an extremely clever man—I still have many of his school prizes—but looking back, I realize that he was a manic depressive and was on occasion pursued by what Sir Winston Churchill graphically described as "the black dog."[11] My father was treated privately and expensively in the 1950s and early 1960s by consultant psychiatrists whom my mother worked hard to pay. My recollection is of individuals using pseudo-science and an authoritarian manner to make money out of other people's distress. I remember to this day how my father was treated with the drug LSD and also with electroconvulsive therapy (ECT)—with machines that, at the time, were so poorly calibrated that no one knew what current or voltage the patient's brain was being subjected to. Tragically, his personality and intellect were permanently shattered, so that he became almost childlike in his behavior. Even now I can remember him begging not to be taken to the clinic for his treatments. Yet at the time, the far more gentle treatment for manic depression based on lithium was available. Had these doctors even heard of the value of lithium for manic depression before they stepped in with their "heroic" solutions? I doubt it. I have since often discussed depression with medical doctors, but none has ever given me what I felt was a rational scientific explanation to justify ECT; indeed, one scientist specializing in brain chemistry likened its use to that of kicking a television to make it work. On the other hand, there is a rational explanation for how lithium helps the brain's "water pump system" clear the brain of "bad" chemicals, thereby helping to lift depression.

At the other end of the scale, the most brilliant, wise, and sensible GP I have ever met was the doctor I've already mentioned (the one I telephoned in the middle of the night from Canada when I first felt a lump in my breast), John Camac. When my mother was first widowed and very lonely and upset, instead of dishing out antidepressants, he bought her a beautiful little dog and visited her every day until she felt able to cope. With his help and support she recovered very quickly. I wonder how many patients would actually be better off with poodles rather than pills? It would certainly make for an unusual prescription!

Your relationship with your doctor, be it your GP or cancer specialist, is crucial to how well you manage the disease. Although it is only natural to be anxious and afraid (and believe me, I was terrified), try to show your doctors that you will work with them to recover your health and that you wish to be fully involved in decisions. It is important that you establish a good relationship with your consultant. You will see later how my unjustified doubts and panic on one occasion probably cost me my breast. Without being rude or aggressive, a woman with breast cancer can involve herself in informed and constructive discussion with her doctors provided she knows the treatment options. That is part of what I aim to do with this book.

How can you quickly tell whether your doctor is going to be a good bet? On page 21 is a quick-and-easy ready reckoner I've produced for you to use: it makes no claim to be scientific, but it will help you focus your mind on the most important issues.

A frequent problem that patients encounter is the use by the medical profession of language that seems calculated to be obscure, even though sometimes it is necessary for accuracy. In fact, more than 2,000 years ago, the Greek physician Hippocrates warned doctors: "Those things which are sacred are to be imparted only to sacred persons; and it is not lawful to impart them to the profane until they have been initiated in the mysteries of the science." Today, too many doctors still seem to be following

A CHECKUP FOR YOUR DOCTOR

Favorable	Unfavorable
Possesses lots of common sense and explains things clearly and effectively	Treats you arrogantly or impatiently and falls back on confusing jargon if questioned
Obviously cares about people	Authoritarian—gets a kick out of telling you what to do, gets angry when you ask questions or suggest what is wrong with you
Demonstrates knowledge that is up-to-date	Demonstrates ignorance of subjects s/he should understand
Technically skillful (e.g., knows how to carry out a thorough physical examination)	Fails to give a thorough examination or to come up with a meaningful diagnosis
Prepared to discuss your health with you on a partnership basis and to recommend dietary, lifestyle, or other changes you can make yourself	Uninterested in underlying cause and displays a clear preference for empirical methods to suppress symptoms; reaches for the prescription pad almost before you have started your second sentence

his advice. Before a medical student can become a doctor, s/he must be initiated into the secrets of a language that, it has been estimated, contains 10,000 new words—words that to most of us seem just as extinct as the Greek or Latin from which they originated.[12] Why, for example, should itching be called "pruritis," a runny nose "rhinorrhea," sneezing "sternutation," or a headache "cephalagia"? These are extreme examples, it is true, but they make a useful point: always insist on fully understanding what your doctor is saying to you, and if s/he starts to use new and alarming-sounding words, make sure you ask for a precise explanation in simpler language. Once you understand the language your doctor is using, clarify any details by asking that s/he draw you a diagram, for instance. Then you will be in a much stronger position to evaluate, influence, and if necessary query your diagnosis and treatment. Once my doctors realized I was a government scientist, they tolerated my questions and tried hard to answer and reassure me. But even then I felt I didn't know enough. It wasn't that they were holding anything back. It's just that their approach seemed so different from mine.

BREAST SELF-EXAMINATION AND AWARENESS

I was angry with myself for not having examined my breasts before. Why had I not followed advice and examined them regularly or had mammography? What should I have done, and what can you do to help yourself?

There is controversy among health professionals about the value of breast screening and early detection, including self-examination. On the one hand, there is the view that early detection significantly improves a woman's chances of survival. On the other hand, some senior doctors point out that by the time a tumor is detected, it may have been developing for several years and will already comprise many thousands of cells, and the outcome will depend on the type and stage of cancer. According to the Breast Cancer Society of Canada (BCSC), the smallest lump usually felt by self-examination is about 1 cm across and contains about one billion cells.

In my own case, however, it was self-examination that saved my life. I had learned what cancer feels like, I know how to examine my breasts, lymph nodes, and liver, and I continue to do this regularly. Each time I had cancer, I was the one who found it, and I sought medical help immediately. Moreover, sometimes my cancer reappeared on a timescale of weeks, so waiting for mammograms or routine checkups would not have helped me. Breast cancer in younger women generally tends to grow faster, which is one of the reasons why more frequent mammography would be required to cut mortality rates in women less than 50 years of age, and that of course would increase the cumulative radiation dose the breasts receive.

The commonsense thing to do is to learn about your body and maintain a regular check on yourself so that you can identify problems as soon as possible and get early medical attention. According to the BCSC, patients with small tumors (less than 2 cm) have five-year survival rates of more than 90 percent, compared with 60 percent for patients with tumors over 5 cm. Also, the sooner cancer is found, the better are the chances for treatment using less drastic methods. If you need help in understanding how to examine your breasts, or other parts of your body, the nurses attached to GPs' offices are generally very knowledgeable and helpful. If their attitude is that you should leave examinations to medically trained professionals and your GP supports this view, then find another doctor.

I have annual physical examinations of my breasts, armpits, lungs, and liver at London's Charing Cross Hospital, and these are available through most GPs that have clinics for women. I recommend that all women over 40 attend a clinic at least once a year. Most breast cancers are found by women themselves (in Canada it has been estimated by the BCSC that nine out of ten breast cancers are found in this way), and teaching self-examination would be far more cost-effective and would expose people to far less radiation than the repeated use of mammograms. In addition, by examining your breasts regularly you learn how they feel normally and you will be able to recognize significant changes and go to your doctor for advice. Initially this may involve doctors in more consultations, but in the long term helping people to understand their bodies and take charge of their own health would save time. In the United Kingdom a helpful breast awareness guide has been produced by Boots the Chemists and the charity Breast Cancer Care.[13] Breast awareness is described as follows: "Every woman should remain aware of her breasts throughout her lifetime. Breast size and shape vary considerably from woman to woman, and so do nipple size and shape. Breast awareness means knowing what is normal for you at all times of your monthly cycle and therefore being able to detect any change which might be unusual for you. Detecting a change early means that any treatments necessary may have a better outcome."

Breast self-examination should start as young as possible so that you learn how your body feels normally, but it becomes more important after the age of 40. It should be done each month at the same time (a few days after your period has ended), continuing even after menopause. The first thing to remember is that most lumps in the breast are *not* cancer.

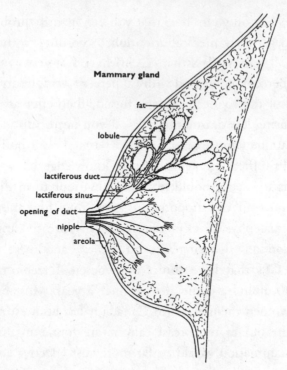

Looking at this simplified drawing of a breast, you will see that each breast consists of fifteen to twenty lobes or segments, each with a duct that opens onto the nipple. Tumors usually develop in the milk sacs or the ducts and, more rarely, in the supporting structures. Most breast cancers are hard and painless, although occasionally they are soft. In carrying out your self-examination try to keep a balanced approach. Prepare to notice changes that may require medical follow-up but remember that they are not necessarily a sign of illness. Nine out of ten breast lumps turn out to be benign or harmless. Here are some useful tips on self-examination:

1. Look at your breasts in a mirror and note any changes in the differences between them. Do this first with your arms by your side, then with your arms raised and your hands cupped at the back of your head. Be alert to any changes in the size or shape of your breasts, any change in the color of the skin, any drawing in of a nipple or pulling in of the skin that looks like a dimple, and

of course any lumps. Lean forward and look at the shape of your breasts from as many angles as possible.

2. Lie down on your back and closely and systematically examine your breast tissue and the tissues in your armpits using the pads of the fingers of your opposite hand. Roll and press the breast area gently but firmly against the chest wall and note any changes, especially hard lumps you have not felt before. Also check for lumps just above the collarbone.

3. Be aware of any bleeding or bloodstained fluid leaking from the nipple. Gently squeeze each nipple to check for discharge.

Remember that although any of these signs can indicate an early cancer, they are more likely to be caused by a noncancerous disease. In any case, if you find any of the symptoms listed above, see your doctor as soon as possible. Even if you are reassured that nothing is wrong, monitor changes and return to the doctor and press for a referral if you think there is a problem. On two occasions I used quantitative measurements to monitor lumps, so I knew what they were doing. I made four tiny marks with indelible black ink at the top and bottom and two sides of the lump, and I used calipers to make measurements, which I recorded on graph paper. I found this very useful on one occasion in convincing my doctor that I had a problem (more about this later). In order to do this, I borrowed the calipers from a colleague who is an expert on fossils.

I am always surprised now when I hear of women—including the late, brave Helen Rollason, who recently died of colon cancer—who have tumors in the liver that are so advanced that the doctor can feel them by simple physical examination, although the women themselves have no idea that they are there. The front lobes of the liver are near the surface of the body just below the rib cage and can be examined easily for obvious lumps. We should all learn the basics of our anatomy and how our body feels normally, and we should examine ourselves regularly to find out when things are wrong—especially when they are seriously wrong. (Indeed, I believe we should be taught self-examination as part of biology lessons at school. Not only would it involve us in making a positive commitment to our own health at an early age, it would make the lessons much more useful and relevant.)

Unfortunately, we have all been persuaded to rely on high-technology methods, which consume lots of resources that some senior doctors believe could be better used elsewhere. If we used breast self-examination more effectively and had annual examinations carried out by nurses attached to GP practices, the resources freed up could be used elsewhere for better cancer treatment. For example, it has been argued that the money could be better spent in using cancer cell cultures from the patient to test the patient's susceptibility to different chemotherapeutic treatments before using them on the patient. This would have the potential for improving the effectiveness of the treatment and reducing unnecessary distress to many breast cancer sufferers.

A TESTING TIME

Before any treatment could be recommended, I underwent a series of tests at Charing Cross Hospital to establish what sort of breast cancer I had and the stage it had reached. The hospital has a specialist breast cancer unit with a team that includes surgeons, radiation therapists, and chemotherapists. Doctors who specialize in breast cancer treatment categorize solid tumors according to the stage they have progressed to. In general, small tumors that have not spread to the lymph nodes or other more distant sites of the body are called stage one tumors; stage two and stage three tumors are more advanced, being larger and involving more lymph nodes. Stage four tumors have progressed to the point of establishing readily detectable secondary cancers (or metastases) elsewhere in the body. The organs breast cancer most commonly spreads to are the lungs, liver, bones, and, more rarely, the brain.

Apart from a thorough physical examination and simple tests which indicated that my blood pressure and urine were normal, I had a mammogram, a needle biopsy, a chest X ray, a liver scan, and a bone scan.

Mammography, which involves X-raying the breast, is by now fairly familiar to most women. In the United States there is growing pressure for women to have annual mammograms after the age of 40. In the United Kingdom mammography is offered on a three-yearly basis as a screening program to women aged 50 through 64. Studies are under way to determine the benefits of screening for women aged 65 through 69.

There is much debate about the value of mammography for early detection especially in younger premenopausal women. Doctors who are opposed to expenditure on it believe that the outcome depends on the nature of the tumor and how aggressive it is rather than on the stage at which it is detected. Mammography works best by detecting small grains of minerals comprising calcium oxalate and/or calcium phosphate that form around cancer cells. The main problem with it is that it depends on using X rays on soft tissues (not broken bones), and in premenopausal women breast density is high. Also, benign lumps may come and go through the monthly cycle and the overall texture of the breast may change, making results difficult to interpret. Mammography therefore throws up some false-positives and a smaller number of false-negatives. Moreover, some doctors have expressed concern about the safety of repeated irradiation of the breasts because the effects of irradiation are thought to be cumulative. There is no good evidence in women younger than 50 that mammography saves lives or alters the course of cancer. Mammography is considered most effective in detecting breast cancer in women between the ages of 50 and 69. In Canada, for example, which has one of the highest rates of breast cancer in the world, it has been estimated that mammography has reduced mortality in the screened population of this age group by 30 percent. Well-conducted mammography thus makes sense for appropriate age groups and for some considered at high risk.

The mammography I underwent was painless although occasionally uncomfortable. The chest X ray was also a painless test to examine my lungs for secondary cancer, and while the liver scan is slightly more complicated, again it was completely painless. Liver scans are based on ultrasound and are similar to the tests used on pregnant women to obtain information about their unborn babies.

The bone scan was more involved and in my case had some entertaining aspects to it. I was first injected with a radioactive substance called technetium in a phosphate compound designed to "stick" to the bones. The radioactive rays given off by the technetium can be detected, and a picture of the skeleton, including irregularities such as tumors, can be built up on a computer screen. I had failed to read the instructions carefully, and between being injected and having the scan I had been to the hospital cafeteria for a cup of tea with the friend who was with me. I did not go to "empty my bladder" as I should have done. During the course of the scan I was struggling to look at the images as they appeared. When the scanner moved to my pelvic area there appeared to be an enormous large luminous mass near what I thought was the base of my spine. Immediately my mind created a fearful image of being in a wheelchair crippled by cancer, until the radiographer's voice said, "You didn't go for a pee, did you?" My bladder was by now full of urine in which the radioactive isotope was concentrated. I was dispatched to the john, and by the time I returned, the "cancer" in my spine had disappeared! After the test I drank several glasses of a well-known cola that contains phosphoric acid to encourage my body to exchange the radioactive phosphates for the nonradioactive phosphate compounds in the cola as soon as possible. (Otherwise, as discussed later, I never drink such products.)

Doctors classify breast cancer into more than a dozen main types, including lobular carcinoma, which originates in the milk-producing glands, and ductal carcinoma, which is one of the commonest types of breast cancer. The results of all the tests established that I had stage one noninvasive ductal carcinoma.

MASTECTOMY OR LUMPECTOMY?

I was finally seen by the surgeon to be given the results of all these tests. Kindly but clearly he described the stage my cancer had reached and reassured me that a lumpectomy followed by radiation therapy would probably clear up the whole problem. He explained that this treatment, which he favored, could increase my chances of a recurrence of breast cancer but did not affect the overall death rate. Put another way, in early breast cancer, long-term survival following lumpectomy and radiation therapy is the same as it is following mastectomy. Hence I stood a chance of keeping my breast but would not be risking my life by doing so.

One of the mistakes I made at this time was to go to see the surgeon alone. I was so distracted by the bad news that I lost several personal possessions. And I was confused about what had been said. The best advice is to take a partner or friend equipped with a notepad and pen.

The surgeon and the other consultants I have seen at Charing Cross

Hospital have always been compassionate but honest, and I prefer this to being given false reassurances.

The mainstays of breast cancer treatment continue to be surgery—lumpectomy (removal of the lump) or mastectomy (removal of the breast); radiation therapy (the use of radioactive rays—usually high-energy X rays—to destroy cancer cells); chemotherapy (the use of chemicals to disrupt the physiology of the cancer cells) or hormone treatments such as tamoxifen, which in certain types of breast cancer (classed as estrogen-dependent) is thought to work by preventing the hormone estrogen from reaching the receptor cells in the cancer or breast tissue cells generally. The problem with some of these treatments (mainly radiation therapy and chemotherapy) is that they can give rise to side effects so harmful that they compromise the benefits of the treatment (in some extreme cases causing other different types of cancer such as leukemia to arise). Also, for reasons that are not understood, they can fail in a significant proportion of cases. Hence doctors can only quote survival statistics to their patients. They cannot offer any assurance of a cure to an individual.

The tests that were carried out on me were used to decide on the best treatment, or combination of treatments, for the type and stage of cancer I had. Since that time, I have talked to many other women who have had breast cancer and I have realized how lucky I was to be treated at Charing Cross Hospital, which is famous for the excellence of its teaching and research. Many women, including some who have been treated privately and expensively, have had doctors who were general surgeons, using an approach that can only be described as in the best tradition of "muddling through," with no attempt to assess the nature and scale of the problem at the outset. It is very important that you be treated by a specialist team such as that at Charing Cross Hospital. Be sure your doctor knows your views, and refuse to be fobbed off with anything less than treatment by a specialist team of excellence. Your life, quite literally, may depend on it. In the case of surgery, for example, be sure you are treated by a surgeon who carries out at least thirty such operations a year, and ask about his or her success rates compared with the national average. Also ask about survival rates generally at the hospital where you are being treated. (Asking for such information is particularly important for men having prostate operations because this operation is more complicated than a mastectomy.) Such statistics need to be treated with caution, however, because some doctors will treat patients whom others regard as incurable. I remember asking senior doctors at Charing Cross at what point they gave up—was it when patients had less than a 50-50 chance of survival? I found their reply very moving. They said that, providing the patient wanted to try to survive, they would never give up.

It was on a Sunday afternoon during the period of waiting for radiation therapy that I made another, and perhaps the most regrettable, of my mistakes. I was suffering badly from premenstrual tension and both my breasts felt sore and lumpy. The more I poked and prodded them, the more I began to imagine I could find tumors everywhere. Finally, in desperation, I rang the hospital. I couldn't see my usual surgeon at such short notice, so I was seen by another doctor. At the time I did not know that the lumpectomy and radiation therapy versus mastectomy controversy was raging within the medical profession. Nor did I realize that doctors on the same team could hold radically different views (although I knew that scientists often do). Anyway, the man who saw me, unlike my usual surgeon, was clearly a mastectomy man. He told me absolutely and unequivocally that my cancer, being noninvasive ductal carcinoma, must be treated by mastectomy. Otherwise, he claimed, I would be dead within three months. He maintained this position under strong pressure and cross-questioning from my husband, who like me is also a scientist. The doctor claimed he had recently completed his studies for a Ph.D. on breast cancer classification, and his recommendation to have a mastectomy was based on his findings—which I later discovered were at odds with the findings of big international studies. (I have always been suspicious of scientists who spend their lives describing and classifying things. I prefer scientists concerned with understanding fundamental processes, and I should have remembered this.) My husband found the doctor totally unconvincing and tried to persuade me to ignore him. I left the consultation stunned and frightened and feeling that for my youngest children's sake (they were 6 and 13 at the time) I had to choose mastectomy.

When I saw my regular surgeon on the next appointment, I was adamant that I must have a mastectomy, although I felt I could not tell him why I had changed my mind. I will never understand why I believed his associate rather than him. Fear and panic induce reactions that can change people's behavior, so the usually rational behave like frightened children. The thing I should have done was to ask for more time to reflect. I do not know, and will always wonder, whether if I had followed the treatment that my own surgeon recommended, my cancer problems would at that point have been at an end.

Mastectomy is the traditional treatment for breast cancer, and the thought of losing a breast is one of the biggest fears associated with the disease. Incidents of breast cancer have been documented back to the early Egyptians, when the principal treatment was cautery, or burning of the diseased tissue. Mastectomy was developed during the Renaissance by Andreas Vesalius, a Flemish anatomist. During the 1800s, surgeons began to keep detailed records of breast cancer patients. Their data showed that even those treated by mastectomy had a high rate of recurrence within eight years, especially when the lymph nodes under the arm were affected. (The importance of observing these lymph nodes was first recognized by a French physician, Dr. LeDran, at the end of the eighteenth century.)

In the nineteenth century, surgeons were committed to radical surgery. The Halsted operation developed in the United States in 1890 was particularly mutilating and involved removal of the breast, armpit, and major chest muscles. When the first practitioners realized that this was not improving patients' chances, they began to remove parts of the shoulder as well. It was not until 1927 that the British surgeon Geoffrey Keynes (brother of the famous economist John Maynard Keynes) first suggested that radical surgery was both cruel and a waste of time. He had deduced that breast cancer, by the time it was detected, had often shed minute cells into the blood supply, and they could have traveled into the rest of the body. Hence, if the cancer had not already become disseminated (metastasized), such mutilations were pointless—and if it had, they were equally pointless.

The debate was still raging in the 1980s when I was treated, although the mastectomy operation used at the time generally involved removal of fewer chest muscles and was less mutilating. One reason for the dominance of mastectomy over lumpectomy was the relatively poor image of radiation therapy compared with surgery, although in France it had long been one of the preferred methods of treatment (perhaps part of Marie Curie's legacy). International clinical trials had already shown that in early breast cancer, lumpectomy followed by radiation therapy had the same lifesaving value as mastectomy. My surgeon clearly knew this, but his colleague at the time was giving out contrary advice based only, it seems to me now, on his own Ph.D. thesis!

Mastectomy still has an important role if the tumor is large in proportion to the breast, in situations where there is more than one primary tumor, or when the breast has many tiny tumors throughout. But none of these situations applied to me.

I think the lesson of this experience is for patients to understand that medical procedures can often be the subject of far more controversy within the medical profession than the public usually realizes. Different specialists may well take opposing views. Quite recently, for example, it became fashionable in the United Kingdom to prescribe cyclotron (machines used for speeding up subatomic particles) treatment for certain cancers (to kill cancer cells by bombarding them with neutrons). Millions of pounds were raised by charities to buy cyclotrons, and even the Prime Minister at the time supported the appeal. Then serious side effects started to be reported. Eventually the Medical Research Council and a number of cancer specialists called for the treatment to be abandoned.[14] Before agreeing to an important procedure, ask these questions:

+ What is the overall success rate for the procedure? (And how is *success* defined?)
+ What is the likely outcome in my own situation?
+ What other therapies are available, and how do they compare?
+ What is the individual success rate of the specialist/surgeon involved?
+ How does this compare with the success rate of other specialists in the same field?
+ What are the side effects (both common and rare)?
+ What is the quality of my life going to be after the procedure?

A good doctor will take the time to answer these questions for you.

I had the mastectomy approximately two weeks later. Physically the operation is not difficult. I talked to my surgeon and my anesthetist well ahead of the operation (standard practice at Charing Cross Hospital) and felt confident in their care for me. Just one thing: at Charing Cross it was standard practice for the surgeon to mark the breast or lump to be removed with a black felt-tip pen while you were fully awake. Although this is disturbing, especially in the case of your breast, just think how much more distressing it would be to wake up from anesthesia and find the wrong bit had been removed. Marking up prior to operations is not standard practice in all hospitals, so if necessary insist that this be done *before* you are given your "premed" or tranquilizer. Before my operation I was given a medication to relieve anxiety, and after counting to ten for the anesthetist I awoke in the recovery room.

Back on the ward I found I had a long line of stitches holding together a scar where my left breast had been and a tube draining from the scar into a bottle that had to accompany me wherever I went; the bottle contained some clear liquid and a trace of blood. The drain is used to prevent massive bruising around the scar. There was relatively little physical discomfort except for my left arm and the back of my left hand, where the drip had been during my operation. After about three days the bottle and drain were removed (this was painless) and after about ten days the stitches were also removed (again this was painless). My surgeon visited me daily and after a few days told me that the pathology report on the breast tissue that had been removed showed no further cancer and that all my lymph nodes were clear. Lymph nodes in the armpit are the body's first line of defense against cancer spreading. Their condition is regarded as the most reliable indicator of the extent to which cancer cells have spread from the primary tumor. This is useful in assessing the stage cancer has reached. More modern methods of assessing lymph node involvement reduce the possibility of a condition known as lymphoedema—painful swellings of the inside of the arm. The condition can be helped, but once it develops it is often incurable.

I was told that on the basis of the pathology report, I should have no further problems and no further treatment was recommended. In the late 1980s when I was treated, preventive or adjuvant chemotherapy, to treat undetected cancer, was rarely used in the United Kingdom. It is used more widely now and is thought to be partly responsible for some recent reduction in U.K. death rates from breast cancer. Research at Oxford University in the 1980s showed that five-year survival rates for women over 50 treated with adjuvant chemotherapy and tamoxifen increased by 25 percent. Such treatments had been introduced about ten years earlier in the United States. Recently, more effective tests have become available to identify those patients who may have undetected cancer and are most likely to benefit from further chemotherapy treatment.

I attended one or two physiotherapy sessions to improve movement in my left arm but then decided to do the exercises myself at my own pace and to suit my own schedule. Others may need the discipline of formal physiotherapy sessions.

DEALING WITH PAIN

I refused, and continue to refuse as far as possible, to take medication prescribed by doctors (including tamoxifen) or available over the counter from pharmacists. Steroids are sometimes given to suppress various types of discomfort associated with cancer or its treatment, but since they depress immune function, I have always refused them. I also try to minimize my use of antibiotics and I cannot remember when I last used painkillers. None of these types of drugs is known to cause cancer, but I just do not like taking man-made chemicals if I can avoid doing so.

I was lucky to have suffered very little pain after surgery. If I had, I would have tried acupuncture rather than chemical painkillers, especially morphine. Acupuncture is said to have originated in China over 4,000 years ago, when it was realized that arrow-wounded soldiers often made surprising recoveries from long-standing illnesses. In 220 B.C. a proclamation was made by the Emperor Houang-Ti (the Yellow Emperor), which read in part:

> I am disturbed by the amounts in taxes and dues that do not reach
> me on account of illness among the people. My wish is that we
> should no longer use medicine that poisons them, or out-of-date
> methods. I want those mysterious metal needles that direct energy,
> to be used instead.

Acupuncture for pain relief is one of the most widely accepted of all complementary medical disciplines. Indeed, the British Medical Association published a report on alternative therapy in 1986, in which it accepted that there is a scientific basis for claims that acupuncture is effective as an analgesic (pain-reliever).[15] Some veterinary surgeons routinely use it to relieve chronic pain in animals. Overall, evidence from randomized controlled trials supports the use of acupuncture in pain conditions including postoperative pain. Such trials also provide evidence of an effect on nausea; hence acupuncture is a potentially valuable method of relieving some of the effects of cancer and cancer treatments, and it does not add to the chemical burden of the body or cause other side effects.[16]

Acupuncture works by stimulating special nerve fibers that inhibit the transmission of other pain impulses to the brain and by stimulating production of the brain's natural painkillers, endorphins—which are capable of closing off pain for long periods of time—and other neurotransmitters such as serotonin. However, some aspects of acupuncture cannot be explained by conventional medicine. For example, changes in the electrical conductivity of acupuncture points associated with a particular organ have been recorded in patients who have conventional diseases of that organ. There are no known anatomic or physiological explanations for these observations. Traditional acupuncturists supplement a detailed case history with observations that are said to give information about the patient's state of health. These include examination of the shape, coating, and color of the tongue; the color of the face; and the strength, rhythm, and quality of the pulse. Both Western and traditional practitioners may palpate to identify points at which pressure causes tenderness or pain. Acupuncture needles are extremely fine and do not hurt in the same way as, say, an injection; patients may even be unaware that a needle has been inserted. Many patients say they find acupuncture relaxing and sedating, though the method does not work well on everybody. If you use acupuncture, it is essential to use only a fully qualified and professionally accredited acupuncturist.

Variations include acupressure, where pressure is applied using studs on elasticized bands to the points traditionally used for acupuncture, and electroacupuncture (EAP), which uses an electrical pulse instead of inserting a needle in the acupuncture point. Lasers are sometimes used now instead of needles. Transcutaneous nerve stimulation (TENS) does not use acupuncture points but stimulates nerves that block pain messages, and it can be used at home. Hypnosis is another option for pain relief that is also thought to work by increasing endorphin production in the brain.*

BREAST REPLACEMENT

Initially I was given a soft piece of nylon filled with plastic wool to serve as a false breast. After about six weeks, when the scar had healed significantly, I attended as an outpatient and was fitted with a well-designed silicone-gel-filled false boob or prosthesis by a caring, helpful woman who specializes in this work. (The earliest prostheses consisted of a cotton bag of birdseed!) Many people are now offered plastic surgery immediately or a short time after mastectomy. I have been offered this several times by Charing Cross Hospital, but somehow I have never found the time. If I do find the time, I shall ask for the operation that uses a muscle from the back rather than silicone or other breast implants. My silicone-gel false breast starts leaking after about two years, and the idea that such sticky material could get into my body is unthinkable. In the meantime, I have come to terms with my false breast. I wear relatively normal bras, and the only special things I buy for my wardrobe are swimsuits that have an inbuilt pouch for my false boob. Wearing the false boob can be uncomfortable in hot, humid weather conditions—especially working in the field as a geologist—although having clean cotton-backed covers helps. But my main problem is losing it! I even left it at Charing Cross Hospital after one of my routine examinations and it had to be posted back to me. The nurses in the breast clinic still tease me about this.

People vary in their openness about breast cancer and mastectomy. I decided to be open but relatively factual and low key about my situation (most people do not want to be "confronted" or overwhelmed by other people's problems). Other breast cancer patients find different ways of coping, and many women do not wish others to know that they have had

---

*For further information on controlling the pain of cancer, including advanced cancer, see the paper by Kathleen M. Foley, *Scientific American,* September 1996.

a mastectomy. They often do not even want people to know they have had breast cancer, in case people assume they have had a mastectomy. These are matters that only individuals and their partners and families can decide for themselves.

THE HALF-TIME SCORE

At this early, crucial stage of treatment, it is worth examining what I did right and what I did wrong, because it may help others in making decisions that are right for them.

What I Did Right
+ Found the strength deep inside—and admitted to myself that there was a problem
+ Sought medical advice as soon as possible and obtained information to calm my fears
+ Made sure that my GP sent me to a specialist hospital, not to a general surgeon
+ Involved my friends and family who were prepared to help, but understood that some were too scared or anxious or frightened to help me at the time (see Chapter 6)
+ Attended for all the tests and followed instructions
+ Listened to people with a positive, supportive approach
+ Tried to remove old wives' tales from my mind and develop a more rational, less scary concept of breast cancer based on scientific understanding (see Chapter 2)

What I Did Wrong
+ Panicked and scared myself by thinking of all the awful things that could happen
+ Listened to people with scary stories
+ Went alone to be given the breast cancer diagnosis instead of taking a partner or friend equipped with a notepad and pen
+ Was too much influenced by a doctor who was not the consultant in charge of my case

If I could revisit this stage in my illness, the one question I would ask would be "Is mastectomy likely to be better than lumpectomy and radiotherapy?" This time I would believe my surgeon, not his colleague.

AN UNWELCOME RETURN

While I was in the hospital I repeatedly asked the doctors and nurses what *caused* breast cancer and if there was any way I could cut my risk of it recurring. Since they kept talking about estrogen (more about this later) I asked if I could be given a diet to help avoid taking extra estrogen in my food or to reduce my own estrogen levels. They seemed to find difficulty with this type of questioning, although I was allowed to talk to a dietician.

The dietician seemed completely bemused by my questions and, although promising to look into the matter, never got back to me and never responded to my phone calls. Overall, the advice was that I should try to forget breast cancer, put the situation behind me, and think positively. The medical professionals at the time appeared to hold the view that they were the experts "in charge" of me and I should not keep worrying myself. I believe they did this with the best of intentions and with the prevailing wisdom that simply thinking positively would help me. (I'm pleased to say that the whole approach seems to be changing for the better now, with increasing efforts made, at least at Charing Cross, to fully inform and involve patients in their treatment.)

But I felt unable to accept the advice. All my training meant that I must have a rational understanding of problems in order to deal with them, and simply trying to put things out of my mind and "think positively" was not something I could do. So I began to read both orthodox and complementary medical texts on the subject and soon discovered references to the work of Dr. Max Gerson and Dr. Alec Forbes (medical doctors), both of whom had produced anticancer diets.[17] Of all the methods available at the time for treating cancer, the idea of changing my diet appeared to make the most sense, so I altered my diet and lifestyle to fit with the recommendations of the Bristol diet book written by Dr.

Forbes.* The Bristol diet is a general anticancer diet. The book describes the elements of good nutrition and recommends eating lots of unprocessed, unrefined foods such as legumes, including peas, beans, cereals, and lentils, and sprouting seeds, with food cooked in ghee (purified butter). Some yogurt and boiled milk is allowed. I told everyone who would listen to me, including my doctors at Charing Cross Hospital, how good this approach was, and despite their skepticism, I believed that I would never have any further problems with breast cancer.

For the next five years, I attended regularly for checkups. But despite maintaining an optimistic attitude, I began to feel uneasy—as if something nasty were bubbling away just under the surface.

I can't say precisely when it first happened, but I began to be increasingly aware of a large, hard lump developing in the scar tissue under my left arm. This was where the drain had been. But whenever I mentioned it to the doctors carrying out my checkups, they reassured me that it was just extra-thick scar tissue. I accepted this, partly because I thought I was living such a healthy lifestyle and following the Bristol diet so religiously that the lump could not possibly be cancer.

But it was.

After my checkup in 1992, I decided to measure the lump and plot its size to decide whether or not I was imagining that it was growing. I used indelible black ink, which I renewed as it wore off, and the sort of calipers that paleontologists use to measure fossils. Early in 1993 when I attended Charing Cross for my checkup I took my plot with me. The lump had grown, although by less than 2 mm in a year. I showed the plot to the young doctor carrying out my routine checkup. I told her my concerns and about the reassurances I had been given. She decided to carry out a needle biopsy. Within days I had been recalled for surgery to remove the lump and two weeks later to remove yet another lump, which was also cancerous, which again I found in the scar tissue. This was the third time I had detected cancer.

There followed a series of tests after surgery, similar to those I had

*The Bristol Cancer Help Centre (BCHC) in Bristol, United Kingdom, now use a diet and lifestyle plan similar to the one described here. People who need individual help with their diet or emotional support can contact the BCHC by telephone at UK 117-980-9505 or by e-mail at info@bristolcancerhelp.org.uk.

when first diagnosed with cancer in 1987. There were no signs that the cancer had spread, and I was recommended to have a course of radiation therapy. I agreed, believing that this would clear what I described to my doctors as my mushroom field for cancer—my left chest wall where my breast had been.

Many people are afraid of radioactivity, and rightly so. It is used a great deal in diagnostic medicine, including mammography, X rays, and bone scans and in radiation therapy. It is worth remembering that according to the U.S. Environmental Protection Agency, about 11 percent of the average dose of ionizing radiation (a particularly damaging type of radiation) received by U.S. citizens is from such medical sources, while less than 0.5 percent is from the nuclear industry. In fact, most (about 80 percent) of the ionizing radiation dose we receive is as gamma rays or alpha particles from radon gas emitted from rocks, soils, and the buildings in which we live and work.

Radiation therapy owes its origins to the first separation of the naturally occurring radioactive isotope radium 226 from a type of uranium ore known as pitchblende, by Marie Curie, who was a student of Henri Bequerel, the person who first discovered radioactivity. Sadly, Marie Curie died of cancer, probably as a result of her exposure to radioactivity during her long years of research, at a time when the dangers of uncontrolled exposure to radioactivity were not appreciated and when safeguards and precautions had not even been thought of, let alone put in place.

Radiation therapy now relies on irradiating cancer with powerful X rays (invisible but very powerful electromagnetic waves of energy) delivered using an externally applied beam, or in some cases by implanting radioactive sources that emit gamma rays (even higher-energy rays). The exact method by which radiation destroys cancer cells is not known, but it is thought either to inflict genetic damage sufficient to kill cells directly or to induce the cells to commit suicide by the process doctors call apoptosis. It relies on the fact that healthy tissues can repair the damage from radiation exposure more readily than cancer cells.

One of the main benefits of radiation therapy is that it can preserve the anatomic structure around the cancer, so it is less mutilating and disfiguring than surgery. Radiation can also destroy microscopic extensions of cancers that surgery can miss and is a safer option for older, frailer patients. Nevertheless, it sometimes fails to eradicate all the cancer cells in tumors, and, like surgery, it is primarily a local treatment. It does not help in cases of stage three or four (metastastic) cancer, except to relieve symptoms. Whole-body radiation exposure sufficient to kill all dispersed cancer cells would destroy tissues vital to life.

In my own case I was treated by powerful X rays created and delivered by a machine called a linear accelerator. When I was referred for radiation therapy at Charing Cross Hospital, I was seen by an excellent consultant radiation therapist who immediately won my confidence because of his meticulous attention to detail in taking my case history and his excellent knowledge of surface anatomy. (I am amazed by how often I have to tell doctors where my lymph nodes are!) He explained clearly and patiently what would happen to me and answered all my questions fully—another sign of a good doctor.

After that I was taken to the treatment room where the angles and intensities for the X-ray beam to be delivered were calculated. The room looked very high tech—like something out of a James Bond movie—but any fear was dispelled by the kind and professional attitude of the radiographers. Tiny black tattoos were made on my skin as reference points. I still have them, but they seem to be unnoticeable unless I specially point them out to people. It was also explained to me that lung tissue is badly affected by radiation therapy and that I would lose approximately 15 percent of my lung capacity as a result of the treatment. (I wonder if smokers realize how limited the options for treating lung cancer are?) About a week later I began treatment. Every day I would check in and sit for a short time chatting to other patients in the waiting room. I would then be asked to change, and a clean white smock would be waiting for me in a cubicle. All clothing and metallic objects must be removed from the area to be irradiated. Finally, I would go into the treatment room. I had to lie flat while a bag of saline was placed where my left breast would have been (I realized that this was done to reproduce the conditions for irradiation following lumpectomy). The machine was then moved into the first position by the radiographer, who left the room but kept talking to me kindly and reassuringly as the beam was delivered. Each time I was treated, my left chest wall area was irradiated using three different positions, which had been designed to remove cancer cells from my chest wall while minimizing radiation damage to my lungs.

Initially the treatment had little or no effect on me, but gradually my skin looked and felt as if I had been very badly sunburned. One is warned against sunbathing after having radiation. To this day, if any sunlight reaches my chest, the edges of the square where I was irradiated reappear. There are many different recommendations for treating the soreness caused by radiation therapy, especially from alternative practitioners, but even herbal remedies contain preservatives that I thought could aggravate my symptoms. In my own case I decided not to use any creams or potions but to maintain a good diet (which was still the Bristol diet) and increase my consumption of foods that contain chemicals similar to those used in the antiradiation pills given to astronauts (more about this later). Also, although I used simple soap on the rest of my body, I washed the burned area in plain water using a low-energy shower. The doctors at Charing Cross were pleased that my skin recovered so well and so quickly after irradiation.

Many people confuse radiation therapy and chemotherapy. They have different side effects. In my own case, apart from the burn in the immediate irradiated area, I had no other problems. I know of no one treated by radiation therapy for breast cancer who lost their hair or felt nauseated (although irradiation of the head or digestive tract for other types of cancer can cause such symptoms). Throughout the radiation therapy I was given blood tests to ensure that I could continue with the treatment. I noticed the regularity with which the equipment was serviced and checked. This is very important, because poorly maintained radiation therapy equipment can be extremely dangerous. I was given thirty-five radiation therapy treatments over a period of seven weeks. At the end of the treatment I was given a thorough physical checkup, repeated six weeks later, which indicated that I was free of cancer. I held a celebration lunch with some of my friends and felt relaxed and happy. This time, we'd really got it beaten.

But then, about six weeks later, on a Friday morning in July, I was chatting to one of my senior colleagues at the British Geological Survey. Idly, I put my right hand on my neck just above my collarbone.

There it was again—a small hard lump in what I knew to be one of my lymph nodes. I knew immediately that the cancer was back.

I can't begin to tell you how I felt. Perhaps you've seen those horror movies in which some supernatural evil killer keeps on returning from the dead to slay his victims. That's an underestimate of what I experienced. Why wouldn't this monster leave me alone? Surely I'd fought it, and defeated it, enough times? But it had come back again—unmistakably cancer. The chill realization hit me that it wasn't going to let me go until it had claimed my life.

I rushed to the telephone and called the consultant radiation therapist's secretary. He returned my call in less than half an hour and explained that even if he saw me immediately there was little he could do because he needed the equipment available at the breast clinic. I was given an appointment for the following Tuesday afternoon. I am sure he knew by examining my neck that it was cancer again, but another needle biopsy was carried out. He reassured me that even if it *was* cancer there were still treatment options available. It certainly didn't feel that way to me.

The lump was subsequently removed at an outpatient surgery at Charing Cross because, although the operation was to remove cancer, it involved only minor surgery. By now I was so emotionally drained that I felt numb about it.

Afterward, it was recommended that I take tamoxifen, but I declined on the basis that I knew it had been linked to increased risk of other types of cancer, such as endometrial (lining of the womb) cancer.[18] Also, I knew several women on tamoxifen who, although putting up with unpleasant side effects, had nevertheless died of their cancer. And at times like that, it is personal perceptions, not statistical data, that we all respond to. I was therefore advised to have my menopause induced by irradiation of my ovaries to remove estrogen and other hormones from my body.

"Ovarian ablation" can be carried out surgically or by using radiation therapy, which is more common now. Mine was to be carried out using radiation therapy. I was more terrified of this than of the radiation therapy I had had for my chest wall. I was particularly worried about having such a rapid menopause and imagined that within a short time I would look much older, with thin skin and gray hair, and that I would develop frail bones. Also, I knew that after menopause most Western women change shape—by a process commonly referred to as "middle-aged spread." This reflects the change in hormone status to one more like that of men, in whom any added weight goes to the waist rather than the boobs or behind, so that postmenopausal women can lose their typical feminine shape. I did begin to experience some hot flashes, but after I started my new diet these stopped. Apparently I do not look postmenopausal because women colleagues at conferences frequently ask me if I have tampons they can borrow, while nurses and doctors doing smear tests or other routine medicals always ask me about my periods. My hair, skin, and nails have actually improved, and my shape is the same as it has been for the past twenty years. I am absolutely convinced that the dietary changes I describe later are responsible for this rejuvenating effect (a clue: most Eastern women manage to stay looking younger far longer than Western women).

About two weeks after the lump's removal, I attended Charing Cross as an outpatient to have the stitches removed. I remember the surgeon confirming casually that the lump had been made up of breast cancer cells, but then he asked me to go over to the mirror in the consulting room. Had he not made a good job? he asked me. Certainly there was hardly a scar to be seen. However, I was not in the mood to congratulate him on his technical skill; instead I was furious at his insensitivity. Did he not realize how devastated I was to know that I had cancer again? Since then, however, I have indeed admired how well the surgeon operated and been grateful that he used cosmetic surgery methods to conceal what could otherwise have been an ugly scar on my neck. I realize in retrospect that he was trying to be kind. Again he gave me a thorough physical examination and declared he could find no trace of cancer.

So that was it, then. No more cancer. By now, every cancerous cell in my body must surely have been cut out or irradiated into nothingness, and my estrogen—supposedly one of the BIG RISK FACTORS—must have been reduced if not removed.

If only that had been true.

About two weeks after the stitches had been removed, and a few days after the treatment to induce my menopause had been completed, I became aware of a large, itchy swelling in the scar. This lump had appeared *in just a few days.* There was pain around it, but the lump itself did not hurt, although it was very obvious. Indeed, it looked like half of a small boiled egg sticking out of the base of my neck. At first I thought it was an infection and was given another appointment with the consultant radiation therapist. When he examined my neck and told me, as kindly and gently as he could, that it was cancer again, I was overwhelmed with foreboding.

Surely there was no hope now. I just wanted to give up. And die immediately. What was the point of going on?

For some reason I thought of the film *Butch Cassidy and the Sundance*

Kid. Toward the end of the film, the two outlaws are pursued relentlessly by a posse of men. Whatever they do to escape, their pursuers just ride on mercilessly in pursuit. That is how I felt: whatever I did to fight my cancer *there was no escape.*

But yet again, the consultant radiation therapist was wonderful. He picked up my mood and spent time persuading me to undergo chemotherapy, despite my protestations that there was no point. (In retrospect I feel guilty for taking up so much of his valuable time.) Finally I agreed that it was worth a try, if only to give me more time with my family, and he arranged that the treatment would begin three days later.

I was very worried about the idea of chemotherapy. I had a mental image of bald, thin people suffering from the side effects of their chemotherapy treatment, which I knew included severe nausea and vomiting. It was the idea of losing all my hair that worried me most. I decided to deal with this by treating myself to a really good wig from a reputable company. One thing I did, which is a simple tip that many people facing chemotherapy find helpful, was to involve my normal hairdresser. He helped me choose a wig of the right color and texture and trimmed it so that it looked almost identical to my normal hairstyle. As it happened, apart from the visit to my hairdresser to have the wig trimmed, I have never worn it because I did not lose any of my hair.

Charing Cross Hospital is famous for the excellence of its chemotherapy department. Chemotherapy involves the administration of anticancer drugs that travel throughout the body via the blood circulation system. Hence it is a systemic anticancer treatment. Many chemical compounds are currently in use, and new ones are constantly being screened and tested. Chemotherapeutic drugs act by preventing cells from multiplying by interfering with their ability to replicate their DNA. In at least some cases, anticancer drugs (as in the case of radiation therapy) are thought to induce suicide or apoptosis of cancer cells. Unfortunately, while the chemotherapeutic agents are in the body they attack all cells undergoing cell division (mitosis). This is why they particularly affect tissues that have a fast turnover of cells, such as the lining of the digestive tract, hair follicles, and bone marrow. This is the reason for the common side effects of chemotherapy, which include nausea and vomiting, loss of hair, and anemia. Damage to the fast-growing cells of the bone marrow can be particularly problematic because, as well as causing anemia, it reduces the ability to fight infections and can increase the potential for internal bleeding because too few red and white blood cells and platelets (the cells responsible for clotting) are produced.

The first chemotherapeutic drugs were developed during the 1940s and were a spin-off of the work carried out by the Nazis to develop methods of chemical warfare. Initially, chemotherapeutic drugs often proved inadequate when administered individually or even in sequence. But during the 1960s doctors discovered that some cancers, such as leukemia, could be cured when several drugs were used in combination. Unfortunately, solid tumors such as breast cancer are only rarely curable with chemotherapy alone.[19]

Just as bacteria develop resistance to antibiotics, some tumors also quite quickly develop resistance to chemotherapy drugs. Indeed, some tumors can develop resistance to several drugs after only one drug has been administered. I was put on a course of treatment based on the drugs methotrexate, fluorouracil, and cyclophosphamide. The first two work by "pretending" to be other substances in the biochemical reactions of cells. For example, methotrexate is chemically similar to folic acid, which is involved in replicating the strands of DNA that carry genetic information during cell division (mitosis). The substitution of methotrexate for folic acid incapacitates the ability of cells to replicate DNA. Cyclophosphamide (which is listed by the National Science Foundation of America as a carcinogen, i.e., a cancer-producing substance) works by actually bonding chemically with particular DNA building blocks, leading to breaks and inappropriate linkages between or within strands of DNA. As in the case of radiation therapy, chemotherapy depends on the ability of normal cells to recover while cancer cells are permanently destroyed because they have lost their DNA "repair kits."

My course of treatment was carried out each Thursday of two consecutive weeks and then I was given a break of about three weeks before being given the next treatment. This was to be repeated for six months, making a total of twelve treatments. In general I was treated extremely well by Charing Cross Hospital and the staff did everything they could to minimize any discomfort or distress associated with the treatment. But it was still grim. In response to my request for an honest appraisal of my chances of survival so that I could plan for my children, try to prepare them for what was to happen, and make arrangements for their future, I was told I probably had three months to live—six months if I was lucky!

Before beginning treatment I was taken through the procedures that would be followed on each day I attended. These began with being weighed and having urine tests and blood tests to ensure that my red and white cell count had not fallen so low that I could not tolerate further treatment. When the results were available I saw a doctor, who then prescribed the chemotherapy drugs on the basis of the results of the tests obtained. I would then go to the hospital pharmacy myself to help the busy staff get the drugs—something which, as you will see below, can be crucial. The drugs were administered in a large open ward full of others being given various chemotherapeutic treatments for a range of different types of cancers. In my case the methotrexate was injected first, and then the other bags of solution were attached to drips and administered through tubes into the veins in the backs of my hands.

There is no getting away from the unpleasantness of the treatment. I felt reasonably well until about four or five hours after leaving the hospital, when I would feel violently sick and would vomit even when there was nothing left to vomit. However, once my antisickness pills were changed to ones that actually block the receptors in the brain that tell you to feel sick, I had much less of a problem and was able to return to work within a couple of days of each treatment.

There was one particularly unfortunate incident in which I was involved later, when I accompanied a friend for her chemotherapy at another hospital. It indicates how important it is to be fully involved if you are to stand the best chance of survival in a busy hospital, however good it is. The doctor took the results of the standard tests carried out before my friend's chemotherapy and entered them into the computer to calculate her drug dosage based on her new weight (the dose is calculated on the basis of your height and weight). When we collected the drugs he had prescribed from the pharmacist, I read the labels (it was second nature for me to do this) and became convinced that the solutions were about *double* the strength they had been on previous occasions, whereas the concentration had been declining slightly as she had lost weight. When I gave the drugs to the nurse in charge of chemotherapy treatment, I told her of my concern and urged her to check the drug doses carefully before giving them to my friend. After about an hour, I went with my friend to see what was happening and, after we promised not to take legal action against the hospital, the nursing sister admitted that the doctor had indeed prescribed about double the strength of chemicals he should have done. Looking at the concentrations in the bags and thinking about the interview with the doctor, I worked out what had happened. The doctor had entered her new weight into the computer where her height should have been.

I did not and do not blame the young doctor concerned. Doctors at breast clinics in any hospital are working under incredible pressure. There should, however, have been a better quality control/quality assurance system in place. For example, the computer should have been programmed to flash a warning and refuse to carry out the calculation of dose under the circumstances (no one could have grown three-and-a-half feet in three weeks!).

When I asked what would have happened to my friend if she had been given the wrong dosage of the anticancer drugs she was being treated with, I was told that it was likely she would have died of liver or kidney failure. I have since heard of several people undergoing chemotherapy dying of liver or kidney failure, though not, I would stress, at Charing Cross hospital. I hope none of them have died because of inadequate quality systems or computer software in the hospitals where they were treated. By the time this happened to my friend, she was following my program and her cancer had disappeared. It would have been ironic if she had been killed by the chemotherapy she no longer needed!

Despite the fact that my cancer disappeared early in my chemotherapy treatment (see Chapter 3), I was persuaded to complete the course, which I did. Apart from sickness, the only minor side effects I had were increased occurrences of cold sores (which I treated with raw garlic) and infections at the base of my nails (which responded to being bathed in warm salty water), reflecting damage to my immune system as a result of the treatment. I also had some abscesses in my teeth, which my dentist treated with special care (because I made sure he was fully aware of the type of treatment I was being given for my cancer). Also, I had horrendous hemorrhoids, or piles, as a result of constipation caused by the antisickness pills I had been prescribed. I soon dealt with those by eating organically grown linseed (also called flaxseed), which is widely available in health food shops and has other benefits in combating cancer (see Chapter 5).

It was during this fifth, final bout with cancer that things really turned round for me. The cancer had gone, not to return. And, also important to me, I hadn't lost my hair. In fact, it became darker and thicker and I attribute this to the new diet and lifestyle I had adopted. Others on chemotherapy who have followed The Plant Program have not lost their hair either. My hairdresser's boss feared that my hair would end up on the floor of the salon, but my hairdresser, David, whom I have known a long time and trusted, believed me when I said I would accept the blame if this happened. He processed my hair as usual: it was permed straight and bleached; it even needed thinning to achieve the same smooth close-to-the-head hairstyle I like. David now actually hands out my diet to other clients who have cancer.

I am not sure exactly how my diet works to prevent hair loss, but I have some ideas. For example, the high content of folic acid it contains would exchange with the folic acid–like methotrexate molecule, speeding up its elimination from the body as soon as it had done its job.

My consultant radiologist (who it was agreed was also my oncologist—or cancer specialist—and remains on my case), while delighted that any sign of my cancer had disappeared by the end of my fifth treatment, was concerned that it would return once the chemotherapy treatment was over. It never has. Seven years later I remain cancer-free. Apparently the drugs I was given at the time were the cheapest standard preparations available, and reading medical textbooks now it is clear to me that it is highly unlikely that they would, on their own, have cured my cancer.

Two years after my recovery, I was offered a new, advanced form of chemotherapy by Charing Cross Hospital. The treatment I was offered this time is, I am told, extremely expensive, but apparently the doctors were impressed by my positive approach and the fact that I had survived much longer than they had expected. They thought they should help me as much as they could. I turned down their offer because I knew that the key to my cure lay elsewhere.

In the following chapters I will tell you why and how I recovered from cancer and, most important, how I remain cancer-free.

Summary of Tips for Coping with Anticancer Treatment

General

1. Insist that you be treated at a hospital with a specialist breast cancer team, which includes a breast surgeon, not just a general surgeon, a radiation therapist, and a chemotherapist.

2. Try to take a partner or friend when you go for consultations with your doctors. Be sure they are equipped with a notebook and pen to take notes. This will minimize confusion and additional stress.

3. If you know you are panicking or feeling emotional, ask your doctors for more time before making irrevocable choices, such as mastectomy versus lumpectomy and radiation therapy. Ensure that you are as calm as possible when you make important decisions or choices.

Diagnosis

4. Listen and read instructions carefully and follow them closely to minimize the need for repeat tests and hence minimize your exposure to radioactivity and other impacts of diagnostic medicine.

5. After having a bone scan, drink cola containing phosphoric acid to try to flush the radioactive agent used for testing from your body as soon as possible. (The agent is usually attached to a phosphate compound so that it will attach to your bones during testing.)

Surgery

6. Before surgery, while you are awake and fully conscious, be sure the breast or lump to be removed is clearly marked with a felt-tip pen by the surgeon who will be operating on you.

Radiation Therapy

7. Wash the affected area with water only—using a low-power shower. Do not use soap or creams—even herbal ones—that could contain irritating preservatives.

8. Eat seaweed, an organic egg a day, and lots of garlic to give your

body cysteinelike chemicals as used, for instance, by astronauts to repair DNA (see Chapter 5).

Chemotherapy

9. Buy a wig with guidance from your regular hairdresser and have him/her style it to your usual hairdo. Drink juices high in folic acid to minimize or prevent hair loss (see Chapter 5).
10. Drink only filtered water that has been boiled to kill organisms that can cause sickness and diarrhea in immunosuppressed patients (see Chapter 5).

2.

Cells Behaving Badly

In this chapter I explain what cancer is the way I wish it had been explained to me when I was first diagnosed with breast cancer. The material is drawn from recently published scientific papers, but it is explained in unscary, everyday language.

When I first told my mother of my illness, she said, "But we've never had anything like *that* in our family!"

At first I was startled by her reaction. Then I remembered that older people—and younger ones, too, sometimes—used to look upon cancer as something shameful: a family secret to be concealed at all costs, like sexually transmitted diseases or mental illness. Instead of saying someone had died of cancer, obituaries often euphemistically said the person had died "after a long illness." Perhaps the reason for this was superstition and fear.

I think a lot of this phobia stemmed from a basic lack of understanding of what cancer is. Even today, most of us still don't seem to understand what cancer is. On one level, cancer is very easy to understand: it is a certain way in which some cells in the body begin to behave badly. What is bad or odd or unusual about the behavior of cancerous cells? Well, normally, parts of your body do not start to grow out of control, do not attack or consume other parts of your body, and do not take off and start up a new colony elsewhere in your body. But cancer cells *do* act in these ways.

In order to understand why cancer is so hard to treat and cure, we need to look at it in a bit more detail and acquire some basic information. If you're tempted to skip this short chapter, let me beg you not to. You're not going to be tested on it afterward, and knowledge is power: if you understand the basic science of cancer, you're in a powerful position to protect yourself, to get involved in your treatment if you ever become a patient, and to play an important role in the increasingly public debate about the number one threat to women's health. As a scientist confronted with the disease, I had to find out as much as possible about what I was dealing with. I found that getting to grips with the most up-to-date facts enabled me to clear my mind of unhelpful old wives' tales, and having a modern understanding of cancer and its treatment helped me to feel less frightened.

WHEN BAD THINGS HAPPEN TO GOOD CELLS

As you probably know, your body is made up of millions and millions of cells living in complex interrelationships with each other. As I've said, usually your cells do not grow out of control, they do not invade each other's territory, and cells from, say, the lining of your intestines or the ducts of your breasts do not take off and start growing in other organs such as your lungs or liver. But it is the property of cancer cells to do precisely these three things that makes them so dangerous.

Even when cancer cells are removed from the human body and grown in a laboratory culture, they behave very differently from normal cells. For example, normal cells are fussy about the nutrients they consume, but cancer cells are not. Also, normal cells reproduce only until they just touch each other, and then they stop (a phenomenon known as contact inhibition). By contrast, cancer cells keep on propagating and will pile up in mounds because they produce a substance called telomerase, which stops them from counting how many times they have reproduced themselves.

So *why* do cancer cells start behaving badly? Why do they grow out of control and eventually, if unchecked, start migrating across the body establishing secondary tumors in a process called metastasis? To understand why, you first need to be aware of the simple fact that your body must make new cells when necessary—and in some tissues that means almost constantly. As your body "wears out," new cells are created to replace older, dead, or damaged ones. This process is called cell division or, more technically, mitosis.

When cells reach a certain critical size and metabolic state, they divide and create new daughter cells. The daughter cell inherits an *exact* replica of the heredity information (an exact replica of the types of genes in an exact sequence) of the parent cell. Not all cells divide at the same rate. For example, liver cells in the adult do not normally divide, but they can be stimulated to do so if part of the liver is removed surgically. On the other hand, the stem cells in human bone marrow are a good example of cells that divide rapidly and almost constantly. The average red blood cell lives only about 120 days. There are about 2.5 trillion of them in an adult body. To maintain this number, about 2.5 million new red blood cells must be produced every second. In total, about 2 trillion cell divisions occur in an adult human every 24 hours; that's about 25 million a second!

Normally, the cells in your body reproduce only when instructed or allowed to do so by the cells around them, according to a complex and highly evolved system that maintains the size and shape of your body throughout your life. Hence your ears and eyes, feet and legs stay in proportion to the rest of your body.

Now you can begin to imagine what can happen if this process goes wrong. If something happens to increase the rate at which one group of cells reproduces, the result will be an ever-increasing number of cells that have no beneficial function to the body, yet are absorbing nutrition at an increasing rate. And that's what a tumor is. If the cells remain in their place of origin and do not directly invade surrounding tissues, the tumor is said to be benign. If the cells invade neighboring tissue and cause distant secondary growths (metastases), the tumor is known as malignant. Because of this ability to invade other parts of the body, the Greek doctor Hippocrates called this abnormal cell process *karkinos,* literally meaning "crab," from which the modern word *cancer* is derived.

THE WRONG KNITTING PATTERN

How can this process go wrong? Well, it's all a matter of control. Cell division, or mitosis, happens according to a well-established cycle. First the cells increase in size and make new proteins before a resting phase; then they make two exact copies of the cell chromosomes. (Chromosomes are the strings of DNA that contain our gene sequence and carry all the instructions about how to make us: blue eyes, freckles, and so on.) Next the chromosomes line up, and finally the cells divide in two. The whole process is designed to make new cells that are exact copies of the ones they are replacing. This sequence of events is controlled by the cell's genes.

Each cell in the human body contains tens of thousands of genes, which provide detailed instructions that determine not only the color of our eyes or hair but also the characteristics of cell division, growth, and death. Genes can be thought of as knitting patterns or computer programs, which in the case of cancer cells have somehow had a few mistakes introduced. Just think how a sweater would turn out of it were made from a pattern with a mistake in it. It's the same idea.

Most cells, no matter what their shape or function, have an outer wall—the cell membrane—inside of which is a thick fluid called cytoplasm. In addition, with the exception of red blood cells, all cells have a "control center" called a cell nucleus. In the cell nucleus are the chromosomes, made of strands of a special substance called DNA that contains our genes. The genes specify how to make particular proteins that carry out their work. When a gene is activated it causes such proteins to be made. Mutations (mistakes in genes) can cause the wrong amounts or types of the protein to be produced, thus sending the wrong message. Then, when the cell begins its cycle of mitosis, there are errors—just like the misshapen sweater made from the misprinted knitting pattern.

Many types of cells, including breast and prostate cells, have receptors. Receptors are special parts of the cell designed to allow particular substances—hormones or growth factors, for instance—to "dock" and deliver their messages. One end of each receptor protrudes into the fluid between the cells; the other end projects into the cell's cytoplasm and in this way creates a conduit along which the message starts to be transmitted. So, for example, when a growth factor "docks" on an appropriate receptor, its message is passed directly into the cytoplasm. There it begins the relay of a message that is carried from one protein to the next until it reaches the cell nucleus. This relay occurs along what is sometimes called a pathway. Once in the cell nucleus, the message activates genes to initiate their instructions—in this case, for the cell to begin its growth cycle. But cells can receive other messages as well.

There are basically three types of genes in normal cells that can go wrong to produce cancer: those that say "grow," called protooncogenes by doctors and researchers; those that say "don't grow," called tumor suppressor genes; and those that say "fix it," instructing the cell to either repair damage or, in extreme situations, self-destruct.[1]

Currently most doctors think that the cells in a cancer are descended from a common ancestral cell that at some point—probably years before any tumor is detected—initiated a program of inappropriate reproduction. Somehow one or more of the "knitting patterns" for the "grow," "don't grow," and "fix it" genes crucial to cell mitosis accumulated a series of mistakes, resulting in the ancestral cancer cell. Normally the body has a complex quality control system to ensure that such errors are detected and eliminated—to the extent of causing damaged cells to self-destruct (apoptosis). But somehow the ancestral cancer cell avoided the body's quality control safeguards and began to grow out of control. Normal DNA repair mechanisms didn't work, and for some reason the body's immune system didn't recognize the cancer cells as abnormal and so failed to kill them off. Even the "final solution" of apoptosis failed to work. You can see from this sequence of events that cancer is actually the result of a series of failures, starting from mistakes in the cell's genes—the knitting patterns.

These mistakes in the genes are called mutations, and most cancers possess mutations in one or more of the three main gene categories.

The first genes that can go wrong are the protooncogenes, the genes that in normal cells produce a series of proteins that relay "grow" messages from receptors outside the cell into the cell nucleus, telling it to grow, develop, and divide. When the genes that make these proteins are damaged, they can cause too much or the wrong types of protein to be produced, thereby instructing the cell to grow inappropriately.

The relay of information between a receptor and a cell nucleus is sometimes called a pathway. When growth factors—present in the fluid between cells—attach to cell receptors, a pathway is activated or "fired"; that is, the relay of the "grow" message is begun. In cancerous cells, the relaying proteins maintain their activity when they should have stopped, or "switched off." In the case of many types of breast cancers, the protooncogenes with the mistakes—those that keep telling the cell to fire' when it should have switched off—are thought to be those that control how the receptors for growth factors behave.

Pharmaceutical companies are currently working on drugs intended to shut down growth factor receptors that have gone wrong and produced breast cancer. Shut-down methods have been shown to work in cultures of cancer cells, but they have not yet been shown to work in the human body. For example, a research team led by Dr. Michael Pollack at the Jewish General Hospital in Montreal, Canada, has shown that insulin-like growth factor (IGF)–binding protein 3 can stop breast cancer cells in culture by regulating the activity of IGF-1, which has been implicated in breast cancer.[2] Research is in progress to formulate a substance that will increase the activity of IGF-binding protein 3 in breast cancer patients, either directly or by stimulating its production in the body. There is more about IGF-1, its role in breast and prostate cancer, and its presence in our diet in Chapter 4.

The second class of genes that can go wrong to produce cancer are called tumor suppressor genes. In normal cells these genes encode for a sequence of proteins to restrict cell growth, induced by cell-to-cell signaling via the fluid between cells—the intercellular fluid. So if a cell is growing out of control, these genes can make a set of proteins to send a different relay of signals to the nucleus. This time it is to say "don't grow." It is the inheritance of mutated forms of the BRCA-1 gene and the BRCA-2 gene (both of which are tumor suppressor genes) that is associated with inherited or familial breast cancer, thought to cause an estimated 5 to 10 percent of all breast cancer cases. Within affected families, the gene can be passed directly from generation to generation, through either the male or the female line. However, not everyone who carries one of the known breast cancer genes goes on to develop cancer. Furthermore, just because a close relative has had breast cancer does not mean that there is genetic breast cancer in your family.

Some researchers have suggested that faults in the BRCA-1 gene are involved in types of breast cancer other than familial (see Robert A. Weinberg in Notes). So presumably the genes can be damaged during an individual's lifetime. Unlike some other cancer genes, which produce proteins that are more unreachable because they are located deep within the cell near the cell nucleus, the proteins that the BRCA-1 genes encode for are secreted into the fluid between cells. In healthy cells, these proteins are thought to be the method by which the breast protects itself against unruly cell division and hence cancer. Further, there is evidence that the same genes responsible for inherited breast cancer may be involved in inherited prostate cancer. According to a Reuters news agency report of 4 August 1999, work by a team led by Dr. D. Easton of the Cancer Research Campaign's Genetic Epidemiology Unit, Cambridge, United Kingdom, has shown that men who carry the mutated BRCA-2 gene are four to five times more likely to get prostate cancer.

It may be important for people to know if they have inherited the mutated forms of the tumor suppressor genes involved in predisposing them to breast (or prostate) cancer.

If you wish to find out whether or not you have inherited faulty genes, you will need to consult an appropriate medical specialist. However, I believe that since the inherited mutated genes implicated in breast cancer are tumor suppressor genes, they are simply failing to "close the barn door after the horse has gone." I believe that changing certain aspects of your diet and lifestyle could help to reduce your individual risk by reducing your exposure to growth factors, as discussed under protooncogenes, above, and hormone and hormone-mimicking substances.

The third group of genes involved in cancer are those controlling the replication and repair of DNA—the "fix it" genes. An example of this type of gene, which is defective in many human cancers, is the p53 gene. The protein that this encodes for has been called the "guardian of the genome";[3] it instructs cells to repair damage and prevents replication of damaged DNA in normal cells. In extreme situation it promotes suicide, or apoptosis, of cells with abnormal DNA. However, when the p53 gene is damaged, it allows cells carrying damaged DNA to survive and replicate so the abnormal cells can pass on and even accumulate their mistakes.

In several types of cancer the genes that have gone wrong encode for proteins deep within the cell. In the case of breast cancer, recent research is hopeful and suggests that the problems are related to proteins responsible for transmitting messages between the cells and intercellular fluid, rather than deep in the cell. This suggests that, in the case of breast cancer, changes in body chemistry, such as those achieved through changes in diet or lifestyle, can help relatively easily and quickly. This is discussed further in Chapters 5 and 6.

ALL IN THE GENES?

Because there is a clear, obvious, and unambiguous genetic component in the causation of cancer, many scientists and laypeople seem to take it for granted that cancer is by definition a genetic disease. Let me explain the way this reasoning runs:

1. Cancer results from genetic errors.
2. Cancer is therefore a genetic disease.
3. There's nothing you can do about your genes, so there's nothing you can do about your risk of getting cancer.
4. The cure for cancer will therefore be a genetic one: spend a few more billions on researching gene therapy and we'll one day find the answer.

This is faulty logic and it is unscientific. Unfortunately, many people who ought to know better seem to believe this mistaken line of reasoning. I do not. According to R. M. Kradjian, M.D., an eminent American breast cancer surgeon and researcher, 80 percent of breast cancer patients have no blood relatives with the disease. Moreover, when one identical twin in America develops breast cancer, the second twin, sharing 100 percent of his/her genes, has less than a 6 percent chance of developing the disease. In the largest study ever conducted of twins, researchers found in the case of breast and prostate cancer that both twins had the disease in between 14 and 30 percent of cases.[4] Researchers in the study assumed that common cancer in twins was solely due to shared genetic defects, but studies of adopted children suggest that environmental factors common to families are also important. All this makes a purely genetic cause for most cases of breast or prostate cancer highly unlikely and indicates that environmental and nutritional factors are far more significant.[5]

Even the term *protooncogenes,* which literally means "first cancer genes" (it is quite a mouthful!), implies that we have genes in our body whose only purpose is to lurk in hiding just waiting for their opportunity to malfunction and cause cancer. In fact, these genes are *essential* for the growth cycle of normal cells. Only *mutated* or *damaged* forms of these genes lead to cancer. But you wouldn't think so from the name. I do not believe that most of those suffering from tobacco- or asbestos-induced lung cancer would be affected if they had not been exposed to cancer-causing agents. And neither do I believe that most of us have genes that will lead us to suffer breast cancer unless we first expose ourselves to something that causes it.

Genetic treatments for cancer are particularly hyped at the moment. These treatments attempt to deliver into the body new, healthy genes or proteins in order to correct faulty genes. But there is concern that gene therapy may be causing deaths. According to Neil Boyce, writing in the *New Scientist* of 13 November 1999:

> Members of the advisory panel that oversees gene therapy in the USA fear that they have not been fully informed following revelations that deaths were not made public. Gene therapists in the USA are supposed to submit reports of deaths and side effects to the National Institutes of Health's Office of Recombinant DNA Activities in Bethesda, Maryland, so that they can be discussed by the Recombinant DNA Advisory Committee (RAC). But some companies have demanded that these reports be kept confidential, while other researchers believed that they did not have to submit reports at all, unless they had evidence that gene therapy caused the death. The Food and Drug Administration will halt a study if it has evidence of harm to patients.

So why does all the research not lead to cures? Probably because all the "new" methods face the same problems and must overcome many of the same obstacles faced by standard chemotherapy. For any method to be effective, it must find, penetrate, and then change or destroy cancer cells without irreparably damaging normal healthy cells.

One of the main results of all the recent scientific research activity has been to show that there are only minimal differences between cancer and normal cells.[6] Only a minute fraction of the tens of thousands of genes in individual cancer cells are damaged and altered. Hence it is extremely difficult to devise treatments against cancer that will not damage normal tissue as much as cancerous tissue.

Cancer treatments may work well in cultures of cancer cells or sometimes in laboratory animals. In the human body, however, not only must the anticancer agent, whether chemical or biological, find the cancer, but it must also find a way to penetrate tumors sufficiently to be effective *without* causing such serious side effects that it cannot be used on human patients. For instance, solid tumors have many barriers to drug delivery: not much blood flows within them, and some agents do not easily diffuse out of the blood vessels into the cancer itself.[7] Also, there are the problems of toxicity, side effects, and the emergence of drug resistance in the tumor cells and immune resistance to foreign proteins in the body generally. Moreover, cancer cells are genetically unstable and can mutate or change so rapidly that they can readily evade recognition by immunology-based treatments and/or rapidly become resistant to many different methods of treatment, including those based on chemicals or gene therapy. Finally, as discussed in Chapter 1, the cost of researching the new methods of treatment is extremely high, and any drugs developed are likely to be so expensive (according to an article in the *Canadian Press and Ottawa Citizen*, 28 July 1999, one new breast cancer drug costs $8,000 for one month's supply) that they are unlikely to be widely available to breast cancer patients—even if they could be made to work in human beings with active breast cancer.

Many new methods of cancer treatment are being developed. They include methods based on gene therapy to correct defective genes (though current procedures fail to deliver genes to a high enough proportion of cells in cancers); molecular medicine aimed at correcting the proteins produced by faulty genes; methods to make cancer cells commit suicide (apoptosis); methods of blocking the formation of small blood vessels to choke off the blood supply that cancers need to grow (angiogenesis inhibitors); and methods to prevent cancer cells from migrating and reattaching to cells in different organs (metastasis). New immunological methods designed to stimulate the body's own immune system into recognizing and destroying cancer cells are also under development. A new drug that has been strongly marketed recently is based on using monoclonal antibodies (these are antibodies produced by fusing antibody-producing cells with special cancer cells to make cells that are able to survive indefinitely) to bind to proteins, called antigens, which are present on all cells. The monoclonal antibodies are created to target a particular antigen or antigens carried on specific cancer cells. One such new drug increases the time to disease progression, for women with advanced breast cancer on chemotherapy, from 4.6 to 7.6 months. Hardly a triumph compared with my survival of seven years due to a simple, low-tech, low-cost approach based on science and common sense.

3.

The Third Strawberry

In this chapter I explain how I used my science, my knowledge, and my experience of working in China and Korea and with scientific colleagues from these countries and Thailand and Japan—as well as a large dollop of good luck—to identify what I believe to be the main factor that promotes breast (and probably prostate) cancer.

Once the panic and fear had subsided after the breast cancer returned for the fifth time, I felt as certain as I ever had been that the only person who could save me was the scientist within.

It was all too clear from what my doctors said, and from reading medical, pharmacological, and chemical textbooks, that chemotherapy treatment alone was unlikely to cure me. For five years I had done everything my doctors had advised and undergone all the treatments they had prescribed. Also, I had followed to the letter the anticancer diet and lifestyle recommended in the famous Bristol diet. Nevertheless, I now had a large hard, cancerous lump in my neck that had grown in only ten days. Clearly, my lymph system was badly affected by breast cancer cells. (Even when cancer cells spread and invade other organs, they retain the characteristics of the organ in which they first developed. So, for example, despite the fact that they may have spread to the lungs, brain, bones, or liver, breast cancer cells and prostate cancer cells remain breast or prostate cancer cells. As you will see later, this knowledge was important to my eventual understanding of how to overcome my illness.)

Years before, I had worked with an American doctor who specialized in multiple sclerosis (MS). At that time, he had described the disease to me as a "slot machine disease." It was a strange expression, and the first time I heard it I asked him what he meant.

"Think Las Vegas," he replied. "You're playing the slot machines. You get one strawberry—no big deal. You get two strawberries in a row—still nothing special. But if you get three strawberries, then you've hit the jackpot big time."

What he was saying is this: if a person had two of the three factors that he thought were implicated in MS (or as he put it more graphically, two strawberries and a lemon) s/he would not develop any symptoms. But in the comparatively rare event of three strawberries coming up, then s/he would have problems—s/he would develop the disease. In the case of MS, my colleague had suggested that the three factors were a genetic predisposition, an infection—and at the time, slow viruses were the fashionable scientific interpretation—and an environmental or lifestyle factor. (My involvement in his work had been an attempt to identify potential environmental factors, particularly in the Orkney Islands and other parts of northern Scotland where the incidence of MS is unusually high.)

Cancer, like MS, can be seen as a multifactorial, multistage disease. This thought gave me my first real glimmer of hope: although there was nothing I could do about whatever might have *initiated* my cancer (probably many years previously), there might be a lot I could do to eliminate whatever was *promoting* it right now.

Since breast cancer develops at different rates over different periods of time in different people, it seemed likely that something in the body maintains an environment that promotes the cancer cells, enabling them to multiply out of control and eventually allowing them to invade other organs in the body. Such a model could also explain why, in some individuals, cancer goes into remission for long periods of time or even fails to recur. On that basis, I had to identify and eliminate that something, that one strawberry, in order to overcome my disease.

Recently I read that eminent epidemiologists from Harvard University[1] distinguish between two different kinds of carcinogens: those that damage genes involved in cell proliferation and migration and those that selectively enhance the growth of cancer cells or their precursors. Looking back I realize that my mission was to find the second kind of carcinogen, something that over a long period of time had been promoting the growth and spread of my breast cancer cells. It would be by removing that factor from my life that I would take out the third strawberry.

So there I was—a scientist about to embark upon the most vital piece of research I had ever faced in my entire life. Like a plot straight out of a nightmare, the deal was starkly, exquisitely terrible: if I got it right, I could have my life back; if not, then it would be the last piece of research I would ever do.

THE SCIENTIST WITHIN

Now, I want to tell you something about myself that greatly benefited me at the time. As an earth and environmental scientist I am trained to observe natural phenomena such as rocks, fossils, volcanoes, and earthquakes and to piece together observations to develop theories to try to understand how Earth and its systems have developed.

Natural scientists like me work in a rather different way from biological and medical scientists. If you think about it, we have to: the timescales of earth processes are so vast (up to thousands of millions of years) that it is impossible to carry out experiments in test tubes or under controlled laboratory conditions as biological scientists do.

Instead, natural scientists work by piecing together fragments of often very sparse information; producing, synthesizing, and refining their theories from observations, observations, and yet more observations. If you remember the tree of knowledge I described in Chapter 1, natural scientists have traditionally worked further up the root system and trunk of the tree than many other disciplines.

This approach has been astonishingly successful. In less than a century and a half, such methods have allowed the amazing story of Earth and the evolution of its life forms to be pieced together. We now know, for example, that Earth was formed about 4,500 million years ago. It has been transformed by a complex interplay of physicochemical and biological processes from a hot ball of dust spinning through space into a planet with a cool and varied surface environment where abundant water and an oxygenated atmosphere are capable of supporting complex and diverse life forms. We also know that the outer layer of Earth is divided into huge plates. These move on million-year timescales in a complex inter-relationship with convection currents deep within the planet, with volcanoes and earthquakes concentrated along the plate margins. Life began more than 3,500 million years ago, since when various diverse life-forms have evolved and become extinct, or survived, in response to changes in environmental conditions.

The findings of natural scientists have often been opposed by scientific orthodoxy. For example, in the second half of the nineteenth century, the famous natural scientist Charles Darwin suggested, on the basis of careful and extensive observations of rocks and fossils in relation to the modern world, that Earth and its life-forms had required more than 3,000 million years to evolve. At the time, Darwin's views were vehemently opposed by many other scientists. Lord Kelvin, in dismissing Darwin's findings, used physical calculations to show that Earth was only 20 million years old. Kelvin was wrong by a factor of approximately 150 times in his calculation—an enormous error for a physicist to make! He made this mistake because he had failed to take account of the heat generated within Earth by its own natural radioactivity. Darwin, the careful observer, was eventually proved right and the orthodox physical scientist was proved wrong.

Later, the Earth scientist Alfred Wegener proposed the then heretical theory that the continents had once formed one large land mass that had split apart to form the present-day oceans and continents. Despite being founded upon careful observation, Wegener's theory was vehemently rubbished by orthodox scientists, who said there could be no mechanism for such a process. Again, as evidence mounted and Wegener's ideas became irrefutable, the theory of plate tectonics finally became widely accepted by the entire scientific community.

More recently, the suggestion of the American scientist Walter Alvarez that there have been mass extinctions of life-forms during the history of Earth (such as the death of the dinosaurs because of the impact of a large meteorite) was ridiculed. Again, this suggestion is now widely accepted by the scientific establishment.

So, having no alternative but to die or find a way out myself, I decided to find a way out. I determined to take control of my situation by using my training as a natural scientist. I would work in the way that had taken me to the top of my career.

I reminded myself that, despite the billions of dollars spent on cancer research worldwide, little had been achieved in combating the upward trend in the global cancer death rate. Despite the dedication of doctors working to treat patients with cancer, the tools that they had at their disposal were essentially the same as those of twenty years ago. If any other area of scientific research had produced so little benefit for such a high cost, it would have been closed down long ago. I would reject the orthodoxy that predicted—on the basis of a classification of the type of cancer I had and the stage it had reached—that I would die in, at most, three to six months. I decided that instead I would look at breast cancer in a detached way as a natural scientist and try to understand the disease as a type of natural phenomenon. I would try to look at it in a holistic way in the tradition of Darwin. This, therefore, was to be my initial approach: look at the facts, the figures, the statistics, the data, and observe, observe, observe.

THE RIGHT HAYSTACK

When you're looking for a needle in a haystack, you must first find your haystack. Sometimes finding the right haystack can be as hard as finding the needle.

That's pretty much how I felt. I knew how I was going to tackle my crisis—by using the techniques of observation that I had been educated in—but where, precisely, should I start looking?

That was the problem. Current thinking at the time was that the factors involved in breast cancer were a genetic predisposition, total life-time exposure to the female hormone estrogen, total animal fat consumption, personality type, and stress. I therefore had five major factors to investigate and, if possible, correctly evaluate. And, of course, not much time in which to do it. Quickly I made preliminary assessments of each factor, as it seemed to apply to me. This is how my initial thinking proceeded.

Genetic Predisposition

The first thing I did was to remind myself that neither my mother nor any of her sisters had had breast cancer (my mother is now 90 and her sister, 93); nor had my maternal grandmother or any of her sisters had cancer. They all lived to a ripe old age. Investigating women in my father's family, a similar story emerged. There was no evidence of any type of cancer in my family. There was therefore no evidence that I was genetically predisposed. Recently it has been shown that inherited mutations of two genes called BRCA-1 (also implicated in ovarian cancer) and BRCA-2 are significant genetic factors in the development of breast cancer.[2] However, only 5 to 10 percent of breast cancers develop because of inherited genetic defects.[3] Inheritance of one mutated copy of a "breast cancer gene" certainly does not guarantee that breast cancer will develop—although every breast cell contains the mutation. Within affected families, the genes can be passed down through the generations through the female or male line. But, as already mentioned, not everyone who carries the gene develops breast cancer. Moreover, the fact that the inherited mutated genes are tumor suppressor genes suggests that if the factors that promote breast cancer could be removed, then breast cancer risk might be reduced even in those with damaged inherited genes (see also p. 58). I decided that, for me, this didn't present a promising line of investigation.

Estrogen

The female hormone estrogen has been implicated in breast cancer since the nineteenth century when a Scottish surgeon, George Beatson, observed that breast tumors regressed in women whose ovaries were removed. Factors thought to increase women's cumulative lifetime exposure to estrogen include early menstruation, delaying childbearing until later life, and late menopause. Some scientists have suggested that increased body weight and the use of birth control and hormone replacement therapy (HRT) pills contribute significantly to estrogen exposure.

It seemed most unlikely to me that a woman's natural estrogen could, on its own, be the main factor in her developing breast cancer. Otherwise why did all pregnant women not develop breast cancer, and why did women, even before HRT was discovered, develop breast cancer long after their menopause, when estrogen levels were greatly reduced? Indeed, the older the woman (and hence the lower the estrogen levels), the higher the risk. It seemed to me, as a natural scientist, more likely that estrogen promotes breast cancer only when another more fundamental factor, or factors, has caused the body's chemistry to malfunction. I decided to look into this in greater detail and discuss it further in the next chapter.

Fat

Many scientists continue to link increased risk of breast cancer to the Western diet and suggest that the factor is total fat consumption, especially the amount of animal fat in the diet, although investigations following up large numbers of women for a dozen years or more have failed to show any clear link.[4] It is now known that the types of fat in different diets vary greatly. For example, Eskimos, who consume large amounts of fat, mainly from whales, fish, and other marine animals, are not subject to increased rates of breast cancer. In my own case, I'd eaten well within official guidelines for fat intake for years, consuming only lean broiled or chopped meat dishes and low-fat cheeses, skim milk, and yogurt. My fat intake, I felt sure, wasn't the factor I was looking for.

Personality Type and Stress

American psychotherapist Lawrence LeShan has suggested that the type of person who internalizes stress is more likely to suffer from cancer. Indeed, he has gone so far as to suggest that there might be a cancer "personality type." (In contrast, aggressive go-getting individuals—the stereotypical personality Type-A people—are more likely to die of heart attacks or strokes.) On the question of stress, I and many other women who have suffered from breast cancer were under stress in our daily lives or indeed had suffered tragic events. However, so have most people—and not everyone develops cancer. Recently, large, well-controlled studies have suggested that there is little evidence to support the widespread belief that emotional factors, whether caused by incidents associated with grief or because of an anxious or depressive personality, cause cancer.[5] Neverthe-less, at the time it seemed to me to be a good idea to develop coping strategies for stress, and this is discussed further in Chapter 6.

Having completed my assessments, I felt that none of the factors, with the exception of stress, seemed to fit my situation. For example, my periods had started late, I had never taken contraceptive or hormone replacement pills, I had given birth to three children and breast-fed each of them, although for different lengths of time, I had consumed very little animal fat, and none of my female ancestors or female relatives had died before the age of 85 and then not of cancer (remember my mother's reaction: "We've never had anything like *that* in our family!").

I felt that somewhere there had to be another factor. And I had to find it.

THE GAME'S AFOOT

"Come, Watson, come!" Sherlock Holmes used to cry when he was on the trail of a particularly exciting case. "The game's afoot. Not a word! Into your clothes and come!"

There's a certain kick you get when you're doing scientific detective work, even when it's a rather grim race against time. Even though I was undergoing chemotherapy and so from time to time feeling desperately sick, I still felt the thrill of the chase as I started to use my brain for my own survival. But I still wasn't sure where to start looking.

Scientists are supposed to be logical, dispassionate types who labor long and hard for their results, but you'd be surprised how many scientific breakthroughs would never have happened without a healthy dollop of good old-fashioned luck. And that's what happened to me.

The first clue to understanding what was promoting my breast cancer came when my husband arrived back from working in China while I was being "plugged in" for a chemotherapy session. He had brought with him cards and letters as well as some amazing herbal suppositories sent by my friends and colleagues in China. The suppositories had been sent to me as a cure for breast cancer. To this day I do not know what they contained, but they looked like firework rockets. I gave them to Charing Cross Hospital for their research, but I was never able to obtain the results. Despite the awfulness of the situation, we both had a good belly laugh and I remember saying that if this was the treatment for breast cancer in China, then it was little wonder that Chinese women do not get the disease!

Those words echoed in my mind. *Why* didn't Chinese women get breast cancer? My mind flashed up the image of an atlas called *The Atlas of Cancer Mortality in the People's Republic of China,* which I had been given by Chinese colleagues when I was working with them a few years earlier. I had been helping to develop a collaborative project between Britain and China, aimed at examining the links between soil chemistry and disease. Specifically, we were examining how low levels of the chemical element selenium might be related to the occurrence of a type of heart disorder called Keshan disease, and also a crippling condition characterized by enlargement and deformity as a result of the degeneration of cartilage called Kashin-Beck disease. Keshan disease is now accepted to be a selenium-responsive endemic condition that mainly affects children and women of childbearing age and that, untreated, results in heart failure and death. Subsequent field trials of selenium supplementation involving thousands of children proved that selenium could effectively prevent Keshan disease.[6]

Initially Western doctors and scientists had been highly skeptical of the findings of the Chinese scientists. It was not until organizations such as the famous Rowett Research Institute of Animal Health in Aberdeen, Scotland, replicated Keshan disease in laboratory animals by feeding them selenium-deficient diets that the findings of the Chinese scientists were accepted. The scientific community, just like the wider community, can often be awfully chauvinistic when it comes to accepting the results of "foreign" scientists. I call this the Raffy syndrome: Refuse to Accept Foreign Facts Yet.

More recently, my own organization, the British Geological Survey (BGS), has worked with Chinese colleagues to develop methods to identify and mitigate the problem of selenium deficiency in crops grown in certain soils, and the incidence and death rates of Keshan in China are now greatly reduced. There is also a greater understanding of the risk factors for Kashin-Beck disease, which include selenium and iodine deficiency in crops. It is perhaps worth emphasizing again that without an understanding of the fundamental *cause* of the problems—which lay in the environment—there would have been little or nothing that conventional Western medicine could have done.

THE NEWS FROM CHINA

The Atlas of Cancer Mortality in the People's Republic of China had always intrigued me. It shows the markedly different distributions of the various types of cancer throughout the country. The distribution of lung cancer, for example, shows the disease to be concentrated mainly in urban areas (consistent with research in the West, which indicates that lung cancer rates in polluted cities exceed those in rural areas, especially among smokers) and locally in areas of tin or uranium mining where inhalation of radioactive aerosols is likely to be a factor. Overall, the mortality rate for stomach cancer in China is high, but the atlas shows that it occurs almost entirely in the cooler, wetter, mountainous areas of the north, while levels are extremely low in the southern tropical areas of the country. This is consistent with the idea that this type of cancer is caused by micro-organisms that grow in food stored for the winter in poor and unhygienic conditions. In contrast, cancer of the nose and mouth is concentrated in south China in a well-defined region behind Hong Kong and Hainan island. The data in the atlas underline the view that cancer is not one disease but many different diseases with different distributions and causes.

What struck me the first time I looked through the atlas was the amazingly low rate of breast cancer shown *throughout* China. The background rate on the map is 1 cancer death in 100,000 women, which is very much lower than rates in the West, which, as already mentioned, approach one in ten women in many countries—a difference of 10,000 times. I knew, however, that data from different countries could not be compared this simply. They must first be converted to fit a model age distribution for the population using a method developed by Professor Sir Richard Doll of Oxford University (the man who first demonstrated the link between smoking and lung cancer). Otherwise, false assumptions might be made. For example, if a type of cancer affects mainly middle-aged and elderly people, as breast and prostate cancer does, and population A has many more young people than population B, then the overall cancer

TABLE 1: AGE-STANDARDIZED (ASR) RATES OF INCIDENCE (PER 100,000)[7]		
PLACE	BREAST CANCER IN FEMALES	PROSTATE CANCER IN MALES
China, Quidong county (rural)	11.2	0.5
China, Shanghai (urban)	26.5	2.3
China, Tianjin (urban)	24.6	1.9
Hong Kong	34.0	7.9
Japan, Hiroshima	33.4	10.9
Japan, Miyagi	31.1	9.0
Japan, Nagasaki	27.1	9.1
Japan, Osaka	24.3	6.8
Japan, Saga	19.1	6.7
Japan, Yamagata	22.7	7.9
England and Wales	68.8	28.0
Scotland	72.7	31.2
Canada	76.8	64.7
United States (white)	90.7	100.8
United States (black)	79.3	137.0

rate would appear to be much lower in population A than in population B—an erroneous impression. Therefore, statisticians have developed a simple method for adjusting data that takes these age differences into account. Data adjusted this way are termed *age-standardized*.

Nevertheless, even using the age-standardized rates of incidence for breast and prostate cancer for China and Japan compiled by the International Agency for Research on Cancer (part of the World Health Organization), the breast cancer rates are *extremely* low compared with those in Western countries (see Table 1).

The age-standardized data show that the lowest breast cancer rates occur in rural China (Qidong county), where only 11 of every 100,000 women contract it (prostate cancer is even lower—0.5 men in every 100,000). The rate doubles in Chinese cities (Shanghai and Tianjin), and at the time I thought this was probably because of the serious urban pollution problem, the severity of which is rapidly overtaking anything the West can produce.

In highly urbanized Hong Kong, the rate trebles to 34 women in

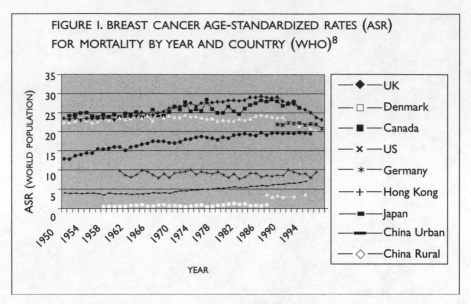

FIGURE 1. BREAST CANCER AGE-STANDARDIZED RATES (ASR) FOR MORTALITY BY YEAR AND COUNTRY (WHO)[8]

every 100,000. The Japanese cities of Hiroshima and Nagasaki have similar rates of breast cancer: and remember, both cities were attacked with nuclear weapons, so in addition to the usual pollution-related cancers, one would also expect to find some radiation-related cases.

The conclusion we can draw from this data strikes you with some force. If you, as a North American woman, were living a Japanese lifestyle in industrialized, irradiated Hiroshima, *you would slash your risk of contracting breast cancer by a half to a third.*

The conclusion is inescapable. Clearly, some lifestyle factor not related to pollution, urbanization, or the environment is seriously increasing the Western woman's chance of contracting breast cancer.

If we expand our view to include other countries, we can see a remarkable picture emerging. The graph labeled Figure 1 (above) shows mortality (deaths) from breast cancer for nine countries. Figure 2 (see p.75) shows the same comparison between countries for prostate cancer.

DECODING THE DATA

Let me just remind you that the statistics we are examining aren't simply the abstract results of some obscure laboratory experiment. They are real-

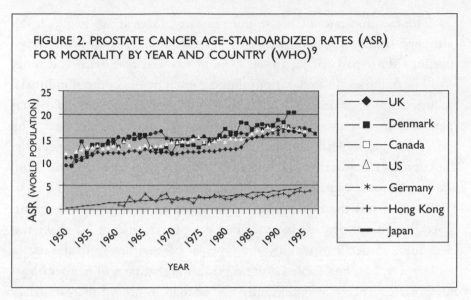

FIGURE 2. PROSTATE CANCER AGE-STANDARDIZED RATES (ASR) FOR MORTALITY BY YEAR AND COUNTRY (WHO)[9]

world, real-life body counts. The knowledge that these studies give us has been obtained at an extraordinarily high price: the neat little graphs reflect the loss of hundreds of thousands of individual lives. The least we can do, as scientists, is to study these figures with all our attention and learn everything we can.

Well, we know first of all that whatever causes the huge difference in breast and prostate cancer rates between Eastern and Western countries, it isn't genetic. Migration studies show that when Chinese or Japanese people move to the West, within one or two generations their rates of incidence and mortality from breast and prostate cancer approach those of their host community.[10] Also, when Eastern people adopt a Western lifestyle in Hong Kong or as some wealthy Chinese do in Malaysia and Singapore, the rates of breast and prostate cancer approach those of the West.

The slang name for breast cancer in China translates as "Rich Woman's Disease." This is because, in China, only the better off can afford to eat what is termed *Hong Kong food*. The Chinese describe all Western food, including everything from ice cream and chocolate bars to spaghetti and feta cheese, as "Hong Kong food" because of the availability of Western food in the former British colony and its scarcity, in the past, in mainland China. This observation suggests that genetic determinants of the disease are less important than environmental factors—suggesting in turn that prevention is possible.

The fact that rates of breast and prostate cancer are so low in Japan (although death rates have risen over the last decade) is particularly significant. Many parts of Japan are as industrialized as Britain and other Western countries. Indeed, serious illness caused by heavy metal industrial pollution was first identified in Japan in the 1950s. For example, Minamata disease, a serious neurological disease, was shown to be caused by eating fish and shellfish contaminated by the industrial release of methyl mercury, and Itai-itai or Ouch-Ouch disease, a painful bone condition, was shown to be caused by eating food contaminated with cadmium. In 1945, Japan was the first country to be attacked with nuclear weapons. Since that time, scientists have studied the cancer rates in Nagasaki and Hiroshima in detail to identify the types of cancers linked to the use of nuclear weapons, but Table 1 (on p. 73) shows that rates of neither breast nor prostate cancer are significantly higher than in other urban centers.

The Japanese environment is in many ways comparable to that of an average Western industrialized nation. Yet the differences in breast cancer mortality rates between the United Kingdom and Japan (Figure 1, p. 74) based on reliable statistical data from the World Health Organization suggest that, despite similar industrial cultures, there is a factor causing a fundamentally different level of risk of breast cancer between the two countries. This observation is also consistent with strikingly similar data from Thailand, China, and other Eastern countries. It therefore seemed a fair bet that the environmental lifestyle factor—the third strawberry— that I was looking for was probably related to a long-standing cultural difference between Eastern and Western countries.

I remember saying to my husband, "Come on, Peter, you have just come back from China. What is it about the Chinese way of life that is so different? Why don't they get breast cancer?"

Over the next couple of weeks Peter and I examined the results of the China–Cornell–Oxford project on nutrition, environment, and health based on national surveys carried out between 1983 and 1984 in the People's Republic of China.[11] The study was led by T. Colin Campbell at Cornell University in the United States, Chen Junshi at the Chinese Academy of Preventive Medicine, Beijing, Li Junyao at the Chinese Academy of Medical Sciences in Beijing, and Richard Peto at Oxford University in the United Kingdom. Eventually the project involved about twenty collaborators around the world analyzing blood and urine samples. The work was carried out in China because it represented a vast laboratory for health investigations, with its huge population living in a wide variety of environments with varied mortality rates from various diseases, different dietary practice patterns, and different socioeconomic conditions.

The China–Cornell–Oxford study established that the Chinese had a higher calorie intake than Americans, but there was much *less* obesity in China; this was attributed in part to higher levels of physical activity among the Chinese and in part to the foods they ate. At the time of the survey, only 14 percent of calories in the average Chinese diet were from fat, compared with almost 36 percent in the West.

So the Chinese ate a low-fat diet: but so did I. The diet I had been living on for years before I contracted breast cancer was very low in fat and high in fiber. In any case, evidence for a simple link between dietary fat intake and breast cancer is at best ambiguous.[12] High total (typically animal) fat intake in adults has not been shown to increase risk for breast cancer in most investigations that have followed large groups of women for up to a dozen years.[13]

Peter and I persevered and discussed the suggestions made by some scientists that it was the high levels of soy consumption in Eastern countries such as Japan and China that gave the female population protection against breast cancer. The soybean is one of the most nutritious legumes known. It has provided the main source of protein in Eastern countries for over 4,000 years. It is used to make soy milk, soy sauce (made by fermenting soybeans), tofu or beancurd (made by coagulating soy with a setting agent such as calcium or magnesium salts), and other products, as well as being eaten raw as beanshoots.

There is good evidence that the soybean contains substances that are cancer-protective. In particular, it is the high content of chemicals called phytoestrogens (chemicals derived from plants, which are closely similar to the female hormone estrogen) in soy that is thought to protect against cancer. These substances are believed to block the effect of estrogen on receptors in breast or breast cancer cells—an effect implicated in the growth of certain types of breast cancers—in a manner similar to that of the antiestrogen drug tamoxifen. Legumes such as peas and beans are plants that fix nitrogen from the atmosphere in the soil. They contain the phytoestrogens called isoflavones. These are also powerful antioxidants, which may also explain their protective effect against cancer. One of the soy isoflavones—genistein—seems to prevent cancer through several means, including by preventing the growth of new blood supply systems (angiogenesis) that cancer needs in order to grow and by inhibiting several key enzymes thought to be included in carcinogenesis. Soy added to the diet of rodents has been shown to decrease the incidence of mammary tumors. Chickpeas—the basis of hummus, eaten throughout the Middle East—as well as lentils and red clover contain a complete range of the isoflavones. Beans, which are the staple foods in some Central and South American countries such as Mexico, also contain isoflavones. Although these populations have breast cancer rates lower than those of the industrialized West, they do not have the exceptionally low rates of China or Japan.

Soy, provided it is organically grown and not genetically modified, is an excellent source of protein that I include in my diet, and it has many other benefits, especially for menopausal women. However, I had been consuming so much soy in various forms, including traditional Chinese bean curd or tofu, that I did not believe it could be the factor I was looking for.

A BELL RINGS

Then one day a couple of weeks later something rather special happened.

Peter and I have worked together so closely over the years that I am not sure which one of us first said, "The Chinese don't eat dairy products!"

It is hard to explain the sudden emotional and mental "buzz" you get when you know you have had an important insight. It's as if you have a lot of pieces of a jigsaw in your mind and suddenly, in a few seconds, they all fall into place and the whole picture is clear. Whenever that has happened to me in the past, I have always been proved right—even if initially my suggestions were regarded as controversial and unlikely.

This is precisely the feeling I experienced. I felt the same buzz, or to use the German-derived word that sums up the feeling so well, *gestalt*. Suddenly I recalled how many Chinese people were lactose-intolerant, how the Chinese people I worked with had always said that milk was only for babies, and how one of my close friends, who is of Chinese origin, always politely turned down the cheese course at dinner parties. I know of no Chinese people who live a traditional Chinese life who ever used cow or other dairy products to feed their babies. The tradition was to use a wet nurse but never, ever dairy products.

Culturally, the Chinese find our Western preoccupation with milk and milk products very strange. I remember entertaining a large delegation of Chinese scientists shortly after the ending of the Cultural Revolution in the 1980s. On advice from the Foreign Office, we had asked the caterer to provide a dessert that contained a lot of ice cream. After inquiring what the dessert consisted of, all of the Chinese including their interpreter politely but firmly refused to eat it and they could not be persuaded to change their minds. At the time we were all delighted and ate extra-large portions!

More recently I attended an international conference in Beijing and was having lunch with two senior Chinese women scientists. A man smelling strongly of spices and garlic walked past, and I suppose my reaction showed. One of my companions giggled and shyly asked me, "What do Chinese people smell of to you?"

I thought about it carefully and replied honestly, "Nothing in particular." Then, deciding that I could legitimately ask the question in reverse, I said, "And what do we Westerners smell of to you?"

There was considerable laughter—usually reflecting embarrassment in Chinese people—but after encouragement on my part, they finally said, "Westerners smell to us of sour milk!"

Of all the Eastern (Chinese, Japanese, Thai, and Korean) cookbooks I have read, none mention dairy products.

THE FINGER POINTS

In my years of exploring alternative health systems—since I first had breast cancer—I have learned that many naturopaths believe that the part of the body that is diseased provides a clue to the cause of the illness. This seems to be particularly the case for cancers of which we know the cause. For example, lung cancers reflect inhalation of cancer-causing cigarette smoke, radioactive aerosols such as the naturally occurring radioactive gas radon, or asbestos dust. Skin cancers frequently reflect excessive exposure to sunlight, and cervical cancer is associated with infection by sexually transmitted human wart (or papilloma) viruses. It seemed highly likely that consuming a powerful biochemical solution from the mammary gland of one species of animal (milk) could be sending the wrong signals to my own mammary glands—my breasts.

And I'd certainly been a big milk drinker. Before I had breast cancer the first time, I had consumed a lot of dairy products as skim milk and particularly as low-fat cheeses and yogurt, which I had used as my main source of protein. I also ate cheap but lean ground beef (which I have since learned was probably often ground-up dairy cow) as hamburgers with my children, especially when we went out for treats, or made it into spaghetti bolognese or other low-cost meat dishes.

At the time of my last recurrence of cancer in the lymph nodes in my neck, I had been eating yogurt and some organic skim milk, which I boiled before drinking, as allowed in the Gerson and Bristol diets. The Bristol diet recommends Indian-style ghee (clarified butter) for cooking, and one of the salad dressings for which a recipe is given is based entirely on yogurt. A detailed case history describing a breast cancer cure in the Bristol diet book also refers to the extensive use of yogurt. I had been careful to choose only those brands of yogurt labeled as "live" and "organic" and I had often made my own yogurt using milk labeled as "organic." In order to cope with the chemotherapy, I had initially been eating organic yogurt as a way of helping my digestive tract recover and repopulate my gut with "good" bacteria.

However, following Peter's and my insight into the Chinese diet, I decided to give up all dairy products immediately. Cheese, butter, milk, and yogurt, and anything else that contained dairy products—it all went down the sink or into the rubbish bin. It is surprising how many products, including commercial soups, cookies, and cakes, contain some form of dairy products. Even many proprietary brands of margarine marketed as soy, sunflower, or olive oil spreads can contain dairy products. I therefore became an avid reader of the small print on food labels. Even many pharmaceutical drugs are in a lactose base, although most medications can be obtained as lactose-free brands.

Recently I discovered that way back in 1989 yogurt had been implicated in ovarian cancer.[14] Dr. Daniel Cramer of Harvard University studied hundreds of women with ovarian cancer and had them record in detail what they normally ate. He compared them with a group of women who were similar in age and other demographic variables but who did not develop cancer. There was one thing that the women with cancer had eaten much more frequently than women without cancer: dairy products, especially the supposedly "healthy" products, such as yogurt.

Dr. Cramer suggested that the culprit might be a normal breakdown product of the milk sugar lactose. Lactose is broken down in the body to another sugar called galactose. In turn, galactose is broken down further by enzymes in the body. According to Dr Cramer, when dairy product consumption exceeds the enzymes' capacity to break down galactose, there is a buildup of galactose in the blood, which may damage a woman's ovaries. Some women have particularly low levels of the enzymes needed to break down galactose, and when they consume dairy products on a regular basis, their risk of ovarian cancer could be triple that of other women. Dr. Cramer observed that the problem was the milk sugar, not the milk fat, so it is *not* solved by using low-fat dairy products. In fact, yogurt and cottage cheese seem to be of most concern because the bacteria used in their production increase the production of galactose from lactose. Although I am not sure that this mechanism explains breast cancer, the link certainly explained my situation and my observations and hypothesis. How I wish Dr Cramer's information had been more widely publicized at the time.

I BECOME A HUMAN GUINEA PIG

Up to this point, I had been steadfastly measuring the progress of my latest and greatest lump with calipers and plotting the results. Despite all the encouraging comments and positive feedback from my doctors and nurses, my own precise observations told me the bitter truth: the first chemotherapy sessions had produced no effect—the lump was still the same size.

Then I eliminated dairy products.

Within days, the lump started to shrink. About two weeks after my second chemotherapy session and one week after I gave up dairy products, the lump in my neck started to itch, and then it began to soften and to reduce in size. The line on the graph, which had shown no change, was now pointing downward as the tumor got smaller and smaller. And, very significantly, I noted that instead of declining exponentially (a graceful curve) as cancer is meant to do, the tumor's decrease in size plotted on a straight line heading off the bottom of the graph, *indicating a cure,* not just suppression or remission of the tumor.

One Saturday afternoon after about six weeks of excluding all dairy products from my diet, I practiced an hour of meditation (more of that later), then felt for what was left of the lump. I could not find it. I went downstairs and asked my husband to feel my neck. He could not find any trace of the lump either. On the following Thursday I was due to be seen by my cancer specialist at Charing Cross Hospital. He examined me thoroughly, especially my neck where the tumor had been. He was initially bemused and then delighted as he said, "But I cannot find it." He was as overjoyed as I was. When I saw the same specialist for my most recent annual checkup (1999), he told me that my chemotherapy treatment had been only the same basic type that has been used for breast cancer for the past twenty years. None of my doctors, it appeared, had expected someone with my type and stage of cancer (which had clearly spread to the lymph system) to have survived, let alone be so hale and hearty.

When I first discussed my ideas with my cancer specialist he was understandably skeptical. But I understand that he now uses maps from *The Atlas of Cancer Mortality in the People's Republic of China* in his lectures and recommends a nondairy diet to his breast cancer patients.

I now believe that the link between dairy products and breast cancer (and probably prostate cancer) is similar to that between smoking and lung cancer. In fact, epidemiological studies have indicated a positive correlation between dairy product consumption and breast cancer risk in publications going back two decades and more. For example, a study in 1970 found low death rates for breast cancer where dairy product consumption was low and intake of other fats was high.[15] Other studies have found a dose-dependent increase in breast cancer risk among women who consumed milk (especially whole milk) and/or cheese. For example, in 1977 scientists examined the incidence of breast cancer in Japan and found a significant increase in both the consumption of dairy products and the occurrence of breast cancer in urban areas where the average intake of other fatty foods was at or below average.[16]

I believe that identifying the link between breast cancer and dairy products, and then developing a diet specifically targeted at maintaining the health of my breast and hormone system, cured me. Initially it was difficult for me, as it may be difficult for you, to accept that a substance as "natural" as milk might have such ominous health implications. In the next chapter, I want to show you some of the factors in dairy products that may be to blame.

4.

Rich Woman's Disease

In this chapter I explain much of the hard scientific evidence that I have collected over the years linking the consumption of dairy products to breast and prostate cancer. I also explain why giving up dairy products is unlikely to cause health problems but is likely to cut your risk of suffering from many other diseases as well as breast or prostate cancer.

Just as many Chinese people giggle in astonishment when they see Westerners consuming such quantities of milk and dairy products, so we find it difficult to understand how anyone could possibly live healthily without them.

It all boils down to a matter of cultural perceptions. To mix metaphors a bit, one person's milk is another person's "yuk!"

In most of Western society, milk is seen as a healthy, natural food: vital for babies, essential for women at risk of osteoporosis, full of protein for hardworking men, a slimming drink for svelte catwalk models. In short, it's all things to all people.

But this carefully crafted image is just that: an image. We have no scientific requirement to consume milk after weaning—in fact, we're the only species that intentionally does so. Even stranger is our obsession with the milk of another species: the cow. It would be just as logical (or indeed, illogical) to drink dogs' milk, pigs' milk, or rats' milk. Those thoughts fill us with disgust. Maybe that's how we ought to feel about cows' milk, too.

Cows' milk isn't intended by nature for consumption by any species other than baby cows. If you compare its nutritional profile with that of human breast milk, you'll see some major differences.[1] The vertical line on Table 2 (p. 86) represents the nutritional profile of human mothers' milk; the horizontal bars show how cows' milk compares, gram for gram. You can see that cows' milk contains about three times as much protein as human milk and far more calcium—both of which may place an excessive burden on young human kidneys. Basically, cows' milk is a perfect food for a rapidly growing baby calf (which gains a bit over 2 pounds or so every day). But that doesn't mean it's good for human babies—or adults!

Many scientists believe that the amount of dairy products in our diet is now far too high. According to the Statistical Abstract of the United States, Americans in 1992 each consumed an average of 564.6 pounds of cows' milk products, or about 1.54 pounds per person per day; this included milk, cream, ice cream, ice milk, buttermilk, cheese, cottage cheese, various dips, and yogurt.[2] The U.S. Department of Agriculture recently estimated that the average American's diet consists of more than 40 percent dairy products, more than double the maximum recommended by any official guidelines. According to Willett and others, the prevalence of obesity in the United States rose by 33 percent between 1980 and 1991.[3]

HOW HORMONES INFLUENCE OUR BREASTS—AND VICE VERSA

The breast is a special gland that develops early in fetal life out of the same type of tissue as the skin.[4] Its structure has been likened to that of a tree, with the tiny sacs in which milk is produced equivalent to leaves, the milk ducts leading from the sacs forming the branches, and the trunk of the tree behind the nipple from which milk is expelled.

As every woman knows, breasts change with age—especially during puberty and menopause and with stages in the menstrual cycle, pregnancy, and sexual arousal. This is because breasts are involved both in bonding with our sexual partners and in feeding and bonding with our babies.

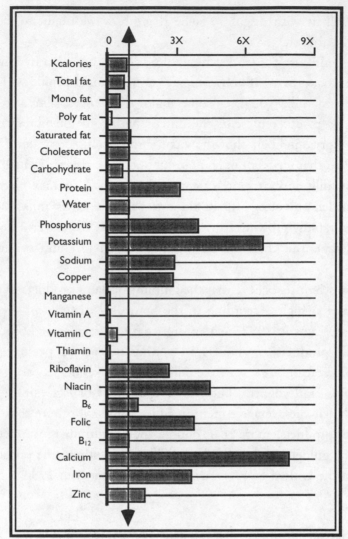

TABLE 2: COMPARISON OF THE COMPOSITION OF TYPICAL COWS'
AND HUMAN MILK (THE VERTICAL LINE REPRESENTS THE
COMPOSITION OF TYPICAL HUMAN MILK)

Breasts can be a source of great pleasure, for example, during sexual activity or breast-feeding children. But at other times they can feel like large, aching, lumpy boils, especially in women affected by premenstrual tension. They can also become a center of disease, the most lethal of which is breast cancer.

Changes in the size, weight, sensitivity, and health of the breasts generally reflect changes in the type and concentration of different chemicals circulating through our bodies. The changes in concentrations of the chemicals can be minute, and only in the past ten to twenty years has it been possible to measure them accurately as a result of advances in analytical methods. The most important chemicals affecting breast function and physiology are chemical messengers, or hormones, which are released in minute quantities, for example, from special parts of the brain or ovaries, in response to biological or physiological factors or outside stimuli. At puberty, growth hormones such as insulin-like growth factor-1 (abbreviated as IGF-1) stimulate breast tissue to develop into breasts. During pregnancy, hormones are also released from the placenta, helping prepare the breast to feed a new baby when it is born. Breast tissue increases, and the milk ducts in the breast sprout extensively under the influence of increasing amounts of estrogen circulating in the blood.[5] As early as five to eight weeks into pregnancy, the quantity and volume of the milk sacs and ducts in the breast have increased so rapidly that the breasts are heavy and enlarged, the nipples are darker, and the superficial veins in the breast become dilated.

Hormones are chemical messengers used to carry information from one part of our body to another. Mammalian hormones have many features in common. They are usually relatively small molecules, and many, such as insulin, are proteins (although testosterone and estrogen are steroids). They are made in endocrine (meaning secreting to the inside) glands, so called because they secrete hormones into blood capillaries within glands for distribution throughout the body via the blood circulation system. The concentrations of hormones in human blood are very small. For any one hormone, the concentration is rarely more than a few micrograms per milliliter of blood, and the rate of secretion is also very low. This is because hormones are so powerful; even the tiny quantities of hormones in our blood can have very large effects on the body.

Each hormone has a particular group of target cells that it affects because they have receptors specific for the hormone. Receptors for protein hormones are on cell surface membranes, and their attachment to the membrane sets off a chain of reactions inside the cell, whereas steroid hormones, which are lipid-soluble, pass into the cell, where their receptors are located.

The interaction of the hormones involved in milk production is par-

ticularly complex. Following the birth of the baby, milk production begins. The breasts first fill with colostrum, a thick yellowish fluid, before
changing to milk as the amount of lactose (milk sugar) increases. (Lactose
is one of the major carbohydrates in milk and is a sugar found only in
milk.) A number of hormones, including prolactin and oxytocin, cortisol,
insulin, thyroid and parathyroid hormones, and growth hormones, enable
this process to commence. Prolactin, in particular, is a key milk-
supporting hormone.[6] The normal levels of this hormone in the blood of
nonpregnant, non-milk-producing women is about 10 ng/ml, but in
breast-feeding women it is two or three times higher. (A nanogram [ng]
is one billionth of a gram.)

Just as hormones profoundly affect every aspect of the breasts' growth
and function, so breast milk itself contains a powerful cocktail of hormones and hormonelike substances. If you have always been used to
thinking of milk as a pure white inert substance full of vitamins, minerals,
and other good things for our bodies to absorb, then you may perhaps
be surprised to think about it in this new way: as a concentrated source
of chemical messengers, each one with a particular mission to accomplish
in influencing the growth and development of the newly born. For example, research indicates that certain components in milk can exert control over aspects of metabolism, including cell division, in the newborn.
Since ancient times, milk has been referred to as "white blood."[7]

Some of the hormones naturally present in milk include oxytocin,
prolactin, adrenal and ovarian steroids, gonadotropin-releasing hormone,
growth hormone-releasing factor, insulin, somatostatin, relaxin, calcitonin
and neurotensin, and prostaglandins (hormonelike substances made in
many parts of the body rather than coming from one organ as do most
hormones), all at levels greater than those in the breast-feeding mother's
blood; and thyrotropin-releasing hormone, thyroid-stimulating hormone,
thyroxine, triiodothyronine, erythropoietin, and bombesin, although these
substances are at lower levels in milk than in maternal blood. Milk also
contains numerous growth factors, including epidermal growth factor
(EGF), insulin-like growth factor (IGF-1), and nerve growth factor. It
also contains over forty enzymes, which have many roles, including the
development of the infant's immunological function and in some cases
the maturation of certain cells.[8]

In fact, all mature breast milk, whether from humans or other mammals, is a medium for transporting hundreds of different chemical components. And it varies in composition between species, between mothers, between breasts, between feeds, and during the course of lactation.[9] Different breast teats have even been shown to produce milk of different composition to suckle different young animals with different nutritional needs.

The point is this: *all* mammalian milk, whether from humans, cows, or other species, is a powerful biochemical solution of great complexity, uniquely designed to provide for the individual needs of young mammals of the same species. It's not that cows' milk isn't a good food: it's a *great* food—for baby cows.

And therein lies the source of the problem.

SOME PROBLEMS WITH MILK

Scientists have linked cows' milk consumption to a wide range of human health problems. Here are some of them:

+ Babies who are fed whole cows' milk in the first year of life are at risk of developing iron deficiency. Indeed, many authorities, including the American Academy of Pediatrics Committee on Nutrition, recommend that whole cows' milk be *excluded* from the diet in the first year of life.[10] The iron in cows' milk isn't easy for babies to absorb, and in addition, cows' milk appears to interfere with the body's absorption of iron from other foods. Even worse, cows' milk has been shown to cause iron loss in babies by producing gastrointestinal bleeding.[11] Pediatricians learned long ago that cows' milk was often a cause of colic in young infants. We now know that breast-feeding mothers can have colicky babies if the mothers are consuming cows' milk, since the cows' antibodies can pass through the mother's bloodstream into her breast milk and to the baby.[12] This is how one British consultant pediatrician describes allergy to cows' milk in infants:

An infant receiving cows' milk protein (CMP) may be persistently restless and unhappy, screaming at intervals and appearing in pain. His appetite may be excessively greedy, he may regurgitate freely and he may have loose, mucousy stools in which blood and sometimes sugars are detected. There may be impaired weight gain and anaemia is common. Infants, especially if their parents or siblings suffer from eczema/hay fever/asthma, may develop facial or generalised eczema, persistent nasal congestion and noisy wheezing when CMP is introduced, or these symptoms may be accentuated at that time, with or without gastrointestinal disturbance.[13]

+ Insulin-dependent diabetes (Type I or childhood-onset) is linked to dairy products. Epidemiological studies of various countries show a strong correlation between the use of dairy products and the incidence of insulin-dependent diabetes.[14] This disease, which tends to strike in early teenage years and accounts for many deaths a year in the United States alone, starts with the immune system destroying the beta cells in the pancreas that produce insulin. There is probably a genetic predisposition, but mounting evidence suggests that the disease is linked to an allergy to bovine (cows') serum protein.

+ Milk is one of the most common causes of food allergies, and it is the *single most common* cause of allergy in infants.[15] Milk proteins, which some people's bodies recognize as foreign proteins, have frequently been implicated in cases of eczema, asthma, and migraine. A meeting of the American Society of Microbiologists suggested that some of the thousands of cases of sudden infant death syndrome (SIDS) occurring in the United States *every year* might be attributed to cows' milk allergy, as babies who are breastfed are less likely to succumb to SIDS.[16] Respiratory problems, canker sores, skin conditions, and other subtle and not-so-subtle allergies can all be caused by dairy products. Over 70 percent of the world's adult population are unable to digest the milk sugar lactose, which has led nutritionists to believe that this is the normal condition for adults, not some sort of deficiency.[17] The symptoms, which include abdominal pain, flatulence, and diarrhea, are relieved by taking the enzyme that breaks down lactose, called lactase. Lactose intolerance may be nature's early warning system: perhaps nature is trying to tell us that we're eating the wrong food!

+ Milk is an excellent culture medium for the growth and transmission of many unpleasant bacteria and microorganisms. Pasteurization was originally developed to destroy *Coxiella burnetii* (the organism responsible for Q fever) and *Mycobacterium tuberculosis* (the organism responsible for tuberculosis), which were thought to be the most heat-resistant pathogens likely to be present in raw milk. However, results of two studies suggest that a microbe called *Mycobacterium paratuberculosis* may survive heat treatment at 145°F for 30 minutes (equivalent to one type of pasteurization) and 161°F for 15 seconds (another type of pasteurization) before it is rapidly cooled to 50°F (equivalent to high-temperature, short-time pasteurization) if it is present in high numbers prior to heat treatment.[18] *Mycobacterium paratuberculosis* causes chronic enteritis in cows, known as Johne's disease, which is an incurable chronic, infectious disease characterized by diarrhea, weight loss, and debilitation. It is one of the most widespread bacterial diseases of domestic animals throughout the world and has been linked to Crohn's disease in humans.[19]

+ *Listeria monocytogenes* is a bacterium that can occur in soft cheeses to such an extent that it causes very serious illness, including meningitis and septicemia; the mortality rate from listeriosis can be as high as 30 percent of those affected.[20] The most vulnerable people are pregnant women and their infants, the elderly, and people who are immunosuppressed, which of course includes those on chemotherapy. These vulnerable groups form a considerable proportion of the population. The incubation period before the development of the disease can be as long as ten weeks, and this causes considerable difficulty in determining the food implicated in the infection.

+ As if this were not bad enough, a wide range of chemicals can be administered legally to dairy animals.[21] These chemicals include antibiotics to treat infection and to promote growth, and antiparasitic drugs including those active against worms. In the United States and some other countries, prostaglandins and pituitary hormones, including oxytocin, luteinizing hormones, and follicle-stimulating hormones, are used as veterinary prescription drugs. It is claimed that their use in cows does not pose human food safety concerns, providing they are used according to label directions. They can, however, be misused—for example, oxytocin can be used to increase milk production—and highly effective policing is needed to ensure that milk does not contain excess residues of hormones administered by dairy farmers.[22]

+ The trend toward intensive farming means that fewer and fewer cows are being unnaturally forced to produce more and more milk (if you thought there was a milk surplus, you're right, but that doesn't have anything to do with the economics of the dairy industry). In the United States, for example, there has been an almost constant annual increase in milk yield per cow of 1.5 to 2 percent. Cows now become pregnant much earlier in their lives, with the shortest possible time between calving. Their young are removed from them, after which they are milked more intensively and for longer periods of time than ever before. Then they are slaughtered. One of the consequences of this highly artificial, high-pressure environment is an increase in mastitis and other infections of cows' udders, which can cause pus to be present in milk. Do you realize that even in the European Union, milk for human consumption can be sold legally even when it contains up to 400,000 somatic pus cells per milliliter? (EU directive 92/46/EEC). So one teaspoon of milk can contain 2 million pus cells. Because increased pus diminishes the value of milk, dairy farmers use antibiotics on their animals. In 1990 a U.S. Food and Drug Administration survey found antibiotics and other drugs in 51 percent of seventy milk samples taken in fourteen cities.[23] There is growing concern that residues such as these may increase the human allergic response to drinking milk, as well as increasing the immunity of bacteria to antibiotics, making human diseases more difficult to treat. It is estimated by the European Union that 3 to 10 percent of the human population is allergic to penicillin and the other antibiotics most commonly used to treat mastitis in cows. Their report also states that increased use of antimicrobial substances in treating mastitis (related to the use of rBGH—see p. 94) might lead to the evolution of resistant bacteria.[24]

+ Milk is designed to be a concentrated source of chemicals that ensure the growth and well-being of newly born and young mammals. Unfortunately, many man-made chemicals that the body cannot distinguish from natural substances *also* become concentrated in milk by the same process. It has been hypothesized that contaminants in milk were implicated in doubling the Israeli breast cancer mortality rate before 1976 (compared with that in other countries with the same average consumption of dietary fat).[25] Three carcinogens found in Israeli milk, one of which was DDT, possess characteristics similar to those of estrogen. Public disapproval of these contaminants resulted in government action in 1978 that drastically reduced their levels in milk. Subsequently there was a decline in Israeli breast cancer deaths. Pollutants such as the fat-soluble PCBs and dioxins, some of which can cause cancer and which are powerful endocrine disrupters, can be particularly concentrated in milk from pasture or feed (see Chapter 6), together with some radioactive isotopes released as a result of nuclear accidents in the past. Recent studies have shown that even breast milk from "clean human beings" has up to 350 artificial chemicals or pollutants in it.[26]

HARD EVIDENCE

We've now seen how cows' milk, although an ideal food for young bovines, is far from ideal for adult humans. But how could dairy products be linked to breast and prostate cancer?

I believe the evidence suggests that consuming dairy products (milk and meat), including low-fat products such as yogurt, does indeed increase the risk of breast and prostate cancer in exposed populations. When I eliminated *all* dairy products from my diet, a large "secondary" tumor comprising cancer cells in the lymph nodes in my neck, which was thought to be incurable, disappeared in weeks. For me, this is pretty compelling evidence.

But that's not all. Since many of the powerful chemicals contained in milk are known to have an important role in the development of young mammals, including cell division, and milk is designed for this purpose, it is worth asking the question: what happens if the chemicals designed to stimulate cell growth in newly born animals send similar signals to adult tissue?

Let's look at some of the suspect chemicals, starting with the previously mentioned growth factor IGF-1. Both insulin and insulin-like growth factors cause cells to increase in size. Insulin has a simple short-term action of cleaning excess nutrients from the circulation and storing them in cells. In contrast, insulin-like growth factors are involved in cell proliferation and differentiation, and a complex set of factors has evolved to ensure that IGF activity occurs only when conditions are optimal for growth. Zinc levels are particularly important in this respect.[27]

In 1994 a genetically engineered copy of natural bovine growth hormone (BGH)* called recombinant bovine growth hormone (rBGH)—also known as bovine somatotropin or BST—was marketed in the United States following approval by the Food and Drug Administration. The hormone is manufactured by taking the specific gene sequence that carries the instructions for making BGH from the DNA of cows and inserting it into *E. coli* bacteria, which are then cultured to produce commercial quantities of rBGH.

The effect of rBGH on the mammary glands of lactating cows is to increase secretory activity, blood flow, nutrient uptake, and milk synthesis. That's what the hormone is supposed to do: when injected into cows it is capable of increasing milk production by an average of 12 percent. There is a moratorium on its use in Europe and Canada, but its use in the United States and several other countries is increasing. For example, between 1995 and 1996 its use increased by 45 percent in the United States alone. Unlike most other hormones used on agricultural animals in the United States, rBGH does not require a veterinary prescription. Under the General Agreement on Tariffs and Trade (GATT), the European Union is unable to ban the import of milk or milk products from rBGH-treated cows from the United States or other countries.[28]

What effect might BGH have in humans? Since it is structurally different by approximately 35 percent from its human equivalent, it is argued that it has no effect because it will be unable to bind to appropriate receptors in human tissues (such as the breast). However, it has also been

---

*Growth hormone or somatotropin is structurally different in different species; therefore it has to be specified as bovine (B) or porcine (pig) (P) or human (H) growth hormone, for example.

suggested by other scientists that the extra amino acids on the genetically modified substance make it exceptionally potent to cows and dangerous to humans.

What is really of concern, however, is what rBGH does to milk. Changes in the composition of milk from rBGH-treated cows were noted as early as 1985 by scientists who reported changes in the proportion of short- and medium-chain fatty acids and of long-chain fatty acids, findings confirmed recently.[29]

One of the most important effects of rBGH, as far as breast and prostate cancer studies are concerned, is that it releases extra quantities of the insulin-like growth factor IGF-1. Insulin and the insulin-like growth factors IGF-1 and IGF-2 are secreted by cells into the bloodstream and intercellular spaces in all mammals. IGF-1 stimulates cell division, especially in the first phase of the cell cycle when the cell enlarges and makes new proteins. It also has insulin-like effects, such as the stimulation of glucose storage in fat cells. The highest proportion of IGF-1 is made by the liver. The liver also makes two proteins that inactivate it—IGF-binding proteins 1 and 3.

Unlike bovine growth hormone, IGF-1 is exactly the same chemical whether it is in the milk of goats, sheep, cows, humans, or other mammalian species. Levels of IGF-1 are naturally higher in cows' milk than in human milk, but its average concentration in milk from cows treated with rBGH is *even higher* (estimates vary from two to five times higher concentration in treated milk), and there is about two times more IGF-1 in the meat of treated cows than in that of untreated cows.[30] Different breeds of cows have different levels of IGF-1. For example, the Brahman breed generally has higher blood levels of IGF-1 than the Angus breed.[31]

Over the years the dairy industry has chosen to increase the average milk yield by selectively breeding from cattle that are better milk producers. This has resulted in the selection of cows that have higher levels of naturally occurring BGH, so that even before the era of rBGH, levels of IGF-1 in milk were increasing anyway. Also, the long-term treatment of cows with the hormone implant estradiol as a growth promoter increases secretion of IGF-1. IGF-1 is not destroyed during pasteurization of milk. In experiments, after being treated at 347°F for 45 seconds (longer than the U.S. Department of Agriculture Pasteurization Protocol), the concentration of IGF-1 was not reduced.[32]

Because IGF-1 is known to be biologically active in humans, causing cells including those of breast tissue in girls during puberty, to divide, the increased levels in milk raises the question: *Will IGF-1 from milk or the meat of dairy animals cause inappropriate cell division and growth and hence cancer in humans?*

In 1998 an American and Canadian research team led by Dr. Susan Hankinson showed that among premenopausal women, those with the highest IGF-1 concentrations in their blood had almost *three times the risk* of developing breast cancer compared to those with the lowest amount of IGF-1.[33] Among women younger than 50, the risk was increased *seven times*! The authors of this study state that there is "substantial indirect evidence of a relation between IGF-1 and the risk of breast cancer" and point to experiments showing that IGF-1 enhances the growth of cancerous breast cells in mice. This study and that of Chan and others[34] into IGF-1 levels and prostate cancer, discussed below, are both prospective studies, whereby symptomless groups of patients are followed for years and data for those who develop disease are compared with data for those who do not. Generally, prospective studies are more convincing for indicating causal relationships than are retrospective studies, carried out when the disease has already developed, in which case there is a chance the disease could be causing the high measured levels of IGF-1.

According to a team led by Dr. M. N. Pollack, Professor of Oncology at McGill University in Montreal, further studies of the association are needed to provide more precise estimates of the effect of IGF-1 on breast cancer and also to investigate the possibility of a relationship between premenopausal levels of IGF-1 and breast cancer in postmenopausal women. The levels of IGF-1 in the blood are highest during the years of puberty, which is, of course, a time of rapid growth. Indeed, at the onset of puberty, IGF-1 signals to breast cells to begin dividing so that the breasts will grow. According to Dr. Pollack, the substance plays the same role in stimulating breast cancer cells. And significantly, one of the ways in which the drug tamoxifen is thought to work is by reducing circulating IGF-1 levels.[35]

Researchers from McGill University and the Harvard School of Public Health have also found increased levels of IGF-1 circulating in the blood to be a strong predictor of prostate cancer.[36] Men with the highest levels of circulating IGF-1 had a 4.3-fold increased risk of developing prostate cancer compared with those with the lowest IGF-1 levels. In the report in the magazine *Science,* Professor Pollack writes that "until now, researchers interested in prostate cancer have focussed on male hormones such as testosterone, but these (IGF-1) results open up a whole new direction of research. This is of the same order of magnitude as the relationship between cholesterol levels and the risk of heart disease."

According to Professor Pollack's team, IGF-1 is a mitogenic (stimulating cell division) and antiapoptotic (preventing cell death or suicide) substance that influences the prolific behavior of many cell types, including certain normal breast cells. Pollack's work is confirmed by another study that also suggests a connection between IGF-1 and prostate cancer risk, finding that men with high levels of IGF-1 in their blood are four times more likely to suffer from prostate cancer than those with lower levels.[37] And yet another recent study from 1998 confirms that increased IGF-1 levels in blood are associated with large relative risks for common cancers.[38] None of these researchers has specifically linked IGF-1 levels in the human body to consumption of milk or dairy products, but in 1996 Dr. Samuel S. Epstein of the University of Illinois in Chicago published a paper arguing that IGF-1 from rBGH-treated cows could indeed promote cancer of the breast and of the colon in humans who drink such milk.[39] Other studies, including that of Outwater and others,[40] which was based on a review of more than 130 peer-reviewed publications, have also suggested such a link.

All this is, in my view, starting to look like a strong prima facie case. In 1995 the European Union successfully opposed approval for the use of rBGH in the EU.[41] Recently a European Commission (EC) committee has confirmed the findings of excess levels of IGF-1 in the milk of cows injected with rBGH.[42] The report of the EU Scientific Committee concludes that the excess levels of IGF-1 pose a serious risk of breast and prostate cancer, stating that "risk characterisation has pointed to an association between circulating IGF-1 levels and an increased relative risk of breast and prostate cancer." The report cites experimental and epidemiological evidence for such an association. It also concludes that the various ways of measuring IGF-1 concentrations and those of its much more potent truncated forms need to be evaluated. It may be, for instance, that available analytic techniques underestimate the actual levels of IGF-1 in milk by neglecting the protein-bound fraction.

While there is still much to be learned about the precise way in which

IGF-1 may be implicated in breast and prostate cancer, we already know enough, in my view, to start to take defensive measures. It has been hypothesized that IGF-1 contributes to breast cancer cell proliferation through actions on IGF-1 receptors,[43] and it has already been shown that:

+ Breast cancer cell cultures respond to minute IGF-1 concentrations by multiplying as much as four- to fivefold.[44]
+ Nearly all breast cancer cell lines (cultures) and breast cancer cells from fresh tumor biopsies have receptors for IGF-1, and binding of IGF-1 to breast tumors is increased compared with normal breast tissue.[45]
+ Median IGF-1 concentrations in primary breast cancers have been found to be significantly higher than in normal breast tissue.[46]
+ IGF-1 also causes changes in the cell cycle and cancer-causing genes, or "oncogenes." Tiny concentrations of IGF-1 alter the relative number of breast cancer cells in each phase of the breast cancer cell cycle.[47] Such alterations may cause the unregulated growth of cancer.
+ Evidence suggests that overexpression of IGF-1 receptors is a key factor in transforming normal breast tissue to breast cancer. In fact, one criterion for the effectiveness of cancer treatments is their ability to successfully lower IGF-1 levels or block IGF-1 receptor binding. Additionally, other hormones and growth factors may interact with IGF-1 in encouraging tumor growth. The problem with IGF-1 may be due to its ability to make transformed cells more responsive to signals from other growth factors.[48]

The argument of the pro-rBGH lobby is that IGF-1 occurs in milk naturally, and that although administration of rBGH to dairy cows increases IGF-1 levels in milk, the levels are within the range of milk from untreated cows, especially those at the stage of early lactation. They also point out that IGF-1 occurs naturally in the human body (but the extent to which the levels reflect the Western dairy-rich diet is not known). However, it would also be true to say that we manufacture our own cholesterol, but cholesterol-related disease (e.g., heart disease) is caused by consuming *extra* amounts of the substance from dairy and other animal products. Could a similar situation not apply in the case of IGF-1? Specifically, that yes, we manufacture our own IGF-1, but could not *disease* be caused by consuming extra quantities of IGF-1 from dairy products and the meat of animals used for dairying? According to Macaulay, although IGF-1 is a normal body component, it may well be associated with malignant disease when present in excess.[49]

In humans, free or circulating IGF-1 levels decline with age, consistent with their role in growth. IGF-1 levels are higher in teenage girls than in teenage boys, and the difference extends into adulthood. Levels are elevated in pregnant women. Although IGF-1 is essential for growth, its levels do not correlate closely with growth rates, suggesting among other possibilities that some IGF-1 may be of external origin. It has been suggested that IGF-1 levels may be affected by nutritional status.[50]

We also know that IGF-1 has growth-promoting effects in response to concentrations as low as 1ng/ml. Milk contains approximately 30 ng/ml, so that two 8-ounce glasses of milk a day would contain 200 ng of IGF-1 per kilogram of body weight per day for a person weighing 70 kg.[51] Also, milk secretions of mammals contain special forms of IGF-1 that are ten times more potent than normal IGF-1. In normal cows' milk, 3 percent of the IGF-1 is reported to be in this form.[52]

Champions of the dairy industry argue that the hormones and other powerful chemicals in milk do not enter the bloodstream because they are destroyed during the digestive process. For example, in the case of rBGH or natural BGH and IGF-1, both of which are proteins, it is argued that they are broken down by enzymes in the digestive tract into simple amino acids prior to absorption. (Hence the need to administer rBGH to cows by injection.) Yet since the early 1990s there have been concerns about the effects of increased IGF-1 levels in milk on the digestive tract. When the National Institutes of Health reviewed the safety of rBGH back in 1991 (concluding that it was safe), it was stated that "further studies will be required to determine whether ingestion of bovine IGF-1 is safe for children, adolescents and adults."[53] They acknowledged that "Whether the additional amount of insulin-like growth factor in milk from [rBGH-treated cows] has a local effect on the esophagus, stomach or intestines is unknown." Three studies suggest a possible link:

+ Some humans suffer from a condition called acromegaly, or gigantism, which is characterized by excessive growth of the head, face, hands, and feet. It is caused by natural overproduction of IGF-1. Importantly, a recent report indicates that people who suffer from acromegaly have an increased incidence of tumors of the colon (a portion of the intestines).[54]

+ Two British researchers, Challacombe and Wheeler, experimented with IGF-1 on human small intestine cells. They reported that IGF-1 promoted cell division (cancer is uncontrolled cell division).[55]

+ A study published in 1995 in the journal *Cancer Research* indicates that IGF-1 promotes the growth of cancer tumors in laboratory animals and in humans by preventing cell death (apoptosis).[56]

Even researchers who support the use of rBGH have admitted that "many more potential effects of ingested IGF-1 on the gastrointestinal tract need to be explored."[57] Certainly the human gut is quite different from that of ruminant animals such as cows, sheep, and goats, from which we obtain dairy products. The digestive tracts of these animals are designed to digest large quantities of vegetable matter such as grass. Moreover, could certain people have digestive tracts that are poorly adapted to the digestion of dairy products because the biologically active chemicals are not broken down and so pass into the bloodstream? Could this "leakiness" of the digestive tract increase under stress? Could it be differences in the ability to digest dairy products that are partly responsible for differences in individual susceptibility to breast or prostate cancer?

One of the arguments of the dairy lobby is that human saliva contains IGF-1, which is known to be broken down during digestion. Independent studies show, however, that growth hormones contained in milk that are closely similar to IGF-1 are *not* destroyed by the digestive system because of the protective effect of casein (the principal protein in milk).[58] The 1999 report of the EU Scientific Committee (see note 52) states "there is clear evidence that orally ingested IGF-1 reaches the receptor sites in the gut in its biologically active form."

Also, it has been suggested that homogenization and other methods of processing milk could increase the risk of cancer-promoting hormones and other chemicals reaching the bloodstream and hence affecting the breast or prostate. Homogenization distributes fat globules through milk so that there are no longer separate milk and cream components. The process involves passing milk through an extremely fine filter at very high pressure to reduce the fat globules (which would otherwise separate out as cream) to about a tenth of their size. By definition, homogenization ensures that the fat molecules are evenly dispersed in the milk so that after 48 hours of storage at 45°F, there is no visible separation of cream. According to some scientists, homogenization encapsulates in fat the biologically active proteins and hormones present in milk (rather the way a gelatine time-release capsule protects cold remedies) until they have passed through the part of the digestive system capable of breaking them down. These hormones would therefore survive digestion and risk being absorbed into the bloodstream. Once in the bloodstream, such chemicals would be able to affect breast and prostate tissue and could also promote cancer cells wherever they have reached—for example, where they occur as secondary tumours in the lungs or liver (remember, breast cancer cells are still breast cancer cells, and prostate cancer cells are still prostate cancer cells). Because of advances in food processing, milk can now be engineered to fit its minimum legal definition, and excess fat, whey, or lactose, for example, can be removed, sold, and added to other food. Hence dairy products now turn up in foods that one would never suspect contained milk-derived components (see Chapter 5).

Breast and prostate cancers have existed in Western populations for a long time. A mid-seventeenth-century painting (see p. 102) by Rembrandt entitled *Bathsheba with the Letter of David* (1654), which hangs in the Louvre in Paris, clearly shows that the model Rembrandt painted had a large tumor in her left breast. Since the time Western populations developed stable farming communities, they have consumed significant quantities of milk, and it is worth remembering that, even without the use of rBGH, milk contains quantities of IGF-1 that have been steadily increasing over the centuries because of the selection of higher-yielding dairy cows. In fact, the recent debate about rBGH may have served mainly to draw the potential problem of IGF-1 in milk—which otherwise only a few specialist scientists would have known about—to the attention of the public.

And yet IGF-1 is only *one* of the powerful chemicals in milk that may have a significant role to play in the development of breast and prostate cancer. What about all the others?

IGF-II

According to Outwater and others,[59] IGF-II is also a potent mitogen (a substance that induces cell division) present in human and cows' milk. The Food and Drug Administration has reported that IGF-1 levels are approximately 30 ng/ml. Those of IGF-II are approximately 350 ng/ml—more than ten times greater. Most studies have concentrated on IGF-1 because of the effects of rBGH on its concentration. One experiment reported by Outwater and others, however, which involved increasing IGF-II levels in transgenic mice twenty- to thirtyfold, indicated the development of a wide range of tumors after eighteen months.

PROLACTIN

The hormone prolactin is a growth factor required for the proliferation and differentiation of the human breast and is a key milk-supporting hormone. Prolactin is found in all milk, although there are differences between human prolactin and that of other species. Prolactin has been linked to breast and prostate cancer by several research groups. For example, Haraguchi and others[60] from the University of South Florida wrote in the *International Journal of Cancer* in 1992: "Prolactin plays a key role in the regulation and growth of mammary cells and influences tumor promotion." Their studies were based on cultures of human ductal carcinoma cells using human prolactin.

Clevenger and others[61] from the University of Pennsylvania, writing in the *American Journal of Pathology* in 1995, concluded that their data suggested a role for prolactin in the pathogenesis of breast cancer. In 1989 Vonderhaar,[62] of the National Cancer Institute, found that the same cell culture responded to the presence of sheep or human prolactin (in the absence of estrogens) with a two- to threefold increase in cancer cell numbers. The second generation of cells produced an even greater response. Vonderhaar concluded that "the data indicates that prolactin alone is a mitogen in human breast cancer cells in long-term culture." Research at the University of Turku, Finland, into prolactin receptors in the prostate has also concluded that prolactin may increase prostate cancer progression because it increases epithelial cell DNA synthesis.[63] Some of the experimental evidence on the ability of bovine (cow) prolactin to stimulate human breast cancer cell cultures is conflicting.[64] The ability of bovine prolactin to act as a mitogen in cultures of rodent breast cancer cells is undisputed, however. According to Vonderhaar, 80 percent of human breast cancer cell lines respond to prolactin as a mitogen.[65] Struman and others in 1999[66] also showed that the human prolactin/growth hormone family are angiogenic—that is, they promote the development of microvascular structures. Remember from Chapter 2 that cancers need to develop a blood supply system, and scientists are trying to develop antiangiogenic substances to effectively starve cancers. The same molecules, however, can have antiangiogenic properties. These properties are thought to be important in the development of the vascular connections between the mother and developing fetus (stress and some drugs, including some for treating psychotic disorders, increase the body's circulating prolactin). Prolactin has also been shown to be a significant driver in breast cancer metastasis by research at the University of Pennsylvania Medical Center.[67]

Most amazingly, in the lab, prolactin is actually measured by adding milk to cultures of a type of cancer cell (rat lymphoma) and weighing the increase in the mass of the cancer to calculate the concentration of prolactin. This technique has been shown to be a sensitive bioassay method (relies on biological rather than chemical reaction) for determining the levels of prolactin in milk, and it *depends upon* prolactin's ability to stimulate cancer cell growth. I actually first discovered this in a book entitled *Breast Feeding: A Guide for the Medical Profession.*[68] Genetically engineered prolactin is also marketed and sold for experiments on prolactin-dependent tumors.[69]

Prolactin in milk has been described as biologically potent, and in suckling infant mammals it influences fluid, sodium, potassium, and calcium transport. Again, we manufacture our own prolactin. Is it not likely that, as in the case of cholesterol, triglycerides, and IGF-1, disease could be caused by consuming foods (especially in large quantities) in which *extra amounts* of this chemical are concentrated? Especially since this is a somewhat different version from that meant to be circulating in the human body.

EGF, CALCIUM, AND PHOSPHORUS

Hence, at least one hormone—IGF-1—contained in milk and the meat from slaughtered dairy cows has been shown to be a cancer promoter. There is evidence that prolactin and IGF-II are also cancer promoters. And these are only three of the many powerful, biologically active chemicals in milk designed to influence development of the newborn of the same species. Epidermal growth factor (EGF), which is also a mitogen (promoting cell division), also occurs in milk. It is well established that EGF stimulates the proliferation of epidermal and epithelial tissues.[70]

In 1998 some fascinating work was carried out at Yale University showing that breast tissues from patients with tumors contained closely associated deposits of calcium oxalate or of calcium phosphate.[71] It is these deposits that are detected by mammograms and indicate the presence of tumors. The deposits have different calcium-to-phosphorus ratios depending on where they occur in the breast. The mineral precipitates associated with tissues near the milk ducts in the breast have calcium-to-phosphorous ratios that are closely similar to those in human breast milk.

Does this suggest that breast tumor cells were trying to produce milk? Had they become malignant and cancerous because some chemicals were telling them to produce milk when other conditions were wrong so that the cells became confused, stressed, and finally made mistakes in copying their own DNA (their own knitting pattern for cell function and behavior)? Could not hormones and growth factors that are derived from food and are circulating in the blood confuse the body's own hormone signaling system?

If breast tissue is frequently bathed in fluid with elevated levels of a growth factor used in nature to signal to females to develop breasts during puberty, and/or a hormone that is the main milk-supporting hormone in lactating animals, it is not surprising that cells make mistakes that can lead to cancer.

ESTROGEN

Officially, exposure to estrogen continues to be considered one of the main risk factors for breast cancer, with testosterone similarly thought to affect prostate cancer. Estrogen is involved in the changes that take place at puberty in girls, such as the growth and development of the vagina, uterus, and fallopian tubes. It causes enlargement of the breasts through growth of ducts, stromal (supporting) tissue, and the accretion of fat. Estrogen contributes to molding of female body contours and maturation of the skeleton. It is responsible for the growth of axillary and pubic hair and pigmentation of the nipples and areolae.

The human menstrual cycle involves the monthly creation of a specially thickened and blood-filled lining in preparation for possible pregnancy. The lining is shed as a vaginal flow of blood if pregnancy does not occur. This cycle of preparation and shedding occurs at approximately monthly intervals. This uterine cycle is under the control of ovarian-secreted hormones, estrogen and progesterone.

Estrogen (from *estrus,* meaning "heat" or "fertility") dominates the first week or so after menstruation, starting the buildup of the special lining of the womb as the ovarian follicles begin their development of a matured ovum. About twelve days after the beginning of the previous menstruation, the rising estrogen (primarily estradiol) level peaks and then tapers off just as the follicle with the egg matures and just before ovulation, when the egg is shed into the womb via the fallopian tubes in preparation for fertilization. Progesterone production, also by special bodies in the ovary, dominates the second half of the menstrual month. The rise of progesterone at the time of ovulation causes a rise of body temperature of about 1 degree Fahrenheit, a finding used to indicate ovulation. If pregnancy does not occur within ten to twelve days after ovulation, estrogen and progesterone levels fall abruptly, triggering the shedding of the accumulated secretory lining of the womb through menstruation, and the cycle begins again. If pregnancy occurs, progesterone production increases, and shedding of the endometrium is prevented, thus preserving the developing embryo. As pregnancy progresses, progesterone production is taken over by the placenta, and its secretion increases gradually to much higher levels, especially during late pregnancy.

Thus the monthly rise and fall of estrogen and progesterone levels explain the events of menstruation and are in turn controlled by other hormones secreted by the master gland—the pituitary gland near the base of the brain.

The whole complex cycle is part of a biofeedback information and control system, with multiple neural centers sharing and integrating many biochemical, hormonal, immunological, and emotional conditions. The system functions as a giant analog computer with the capacity to formulate and send chemical messages (hormones) to the pituitary, as well as to control many other body functions, including our immune system and our emotional well-being. It is no wonder that menstruation (and a great number of other body functions) can be affected by diet, emotional states of mind, stress, other hormones, illness, or drugs of all sorts.

Progesterone and estrogen are closely interrelated in many ways. Progesterone is a precursor of estrogen. The three most important hormones of the estrogen class are estrone, estradiol, and estriol. In popular writing, however, each of the specific members of the class continues to be referred to as estrogen. In the case of progesterone, only a single hormone is found. Thus progesterone is the name of both the class and the single member of the class.

The word *estrogen* generally refers to the class of hormones produced by the body with somewhat similar estruslike actions. Phytoestrogens refer to plant compounds with estrogen-like activity. The three main groups of dietary phytoestrogens are isoflavones (enriched in soybeans), coumestans (clover and alfalfa sprouts), and lignans (oil seeds such as flaxseed). Xenoestrogens (literally "stranger estrogens") are other man-made chemical compounds (usually derived from petrochemicals) with estrogen-like activity. Some of the xenoestrogens are very potent estrogenic compounds even in extremely small doses. They are discussed in the section on endocrine-disrupting chemicals in Chapter 6.

Because estrone is generally synthesized first, it is referred to as E_1, estradiol as E_2, and estriol as E_3. In nonpregnant women, E_1 and E_2 are produced by the ovary in relatively large quantities and E_3 is only a scant by-product of E_1 metabolism. Relative serum E_1 and E_2 levels are determined mainly by the activity of the liver, which can convert one into the other, resulting in higher levels of E_2.

During pregnancy, however, the placenta is the major source of estrogens; E_3 is produced in higher quantities, while E_1 and E_2 are produced in lesser amounts. The placenta also becomes the major source of progesterone, producing relatively large quantities, especially during late pregnancy. Estriol (E_3) and progesterone are the major sex steroids (fat-based hormones) during pregnancy. Both estriol and progesterone are essentially devoid of the ability to affect secondary sex characteristics, and thus the sexual development of the fetus should be determined solely by its own DNA and not the sex hormones of the mother.

Among the three estrogens, estradiol (E_2) is the most stimulating to the breast and estriol (E_3) is the least, their relative ratio of activity being 1,000 to 1. Studies of two decades ago found estradiol (and estrone to a lesser extent) to increase one's risk of breast cancer, whereas estriol is protective.[72]

Dairy milk does contain estrogen (and testosterone), although it has been suggested that the levels are so low that cows' milk estrogen is biologically insignificant.[73] Yet for some chemicals, even *very* low levels can cause severe biological damage (just remember what the tiny changes in our own hormones do to our breasts during the normal menstrual cycle, for example). One illustration of this was the problem caused by the effects of a chemical called tributyl tin on dog whelks on Britain's south coast. The chemical was developed for use in paint to coat the underside of ships to prevent the growth of creatures such as barnacles that increase friction and thus slow ships down. The levels of tributyl tin in water were only of the order of five parts in a millionth of a millionth of seawater and were barely detectable. Nevertheless, in the 1980s, over a wide area of Britain's south coast, where minute traces of the chemical occurred, female dog whelks died as a result of their egg tubes becoming blocked by their own eggs because they had developed male organs that had overgrown their female organs. It is difficult to comprehend how such an infinitesimal amount of a substance in the open sea could have such a profound effect, but it did. Unfortunately, the chemical is still licensed for use on larger ships, including those used by the Royal Navy, and is accumulating in some of Britain's offshore sediments to levels well above those known to cause problems in vulnerable marine organisms.

According to three senior American medical researchers, Outwater and others, although estrogens in milk may or may not exert a direct effect, they may stimulate expression of IGF-1, resulting in indirect long-term tumor growth.[74] Free estrogens have been found in commercial pasteurized whole cows' milk, and although their levels are lower, they are still present in skim milk. These authors suggest that the correlation between estrogen levels and milk fat may offer a partial explanation of why, in some epidemiological studies, breast cancer has been correlated with high-fat diets containing dairy products.

The Royal Society, Britain's most prestigious scientific body, equivalent to the U.S. National Academy of Sciences, has recently published a report on endocrine-disrupting chemicals in which it is stated that "Increased consumption of dairy produce may have altered exposure to estrogens." They also state that "Dairy practices have changed this century such that pregnant cows (which produce high levels of estrogen) continue to be milked. Significant levels of conjugated estrogens are therefore present in cows' milk. The extent to which these conjugated estrogens are activated in the human gut and how much estrogen the consumer would then be exposed to is largely unknown."[75]

Let me finish by quoting from the final conclusions of the review paper by Outwater and others who studied the findings of about 130 peer-reviewed publications:

> The existing evidence indicates possible cancer risks associated with the consumption of dairy products. Bovine GH has not been considered to be of health concern because subsequent increase in bovine milk IGF-1 levels are within the "normal range" based on untreated cows' and human breast milk. However, it is possible that the "nor-

mal range" could be carcinogenic when milk is ingested regularly over a lifetime. Hormones and growth factors in milk, such as IGF-1, are consumed in nature by the fast-growing infant; it may be that regular milk ingestion after the age of weaning produces enough IGF-1 in mammary tissue to cause the cell cycle to supercede its boundaries of control, increasing the risk of cancer.

This same point is also made by the EU Scientific Committee on Veterinary Measures Relating to Public Health.[76] They state, "The physiological actions of IGF-1 and IGF-2 relate to growth and development of the embryo and fetus and to cellular differentiation, proliferation and cancer." Is this not just a modern, high-technology way of saying what the Chinese have always known: that milk is just for babies?

In Summary

This chapter has presented you with a lot of scientific evidence drawn from peer-reviewed scientific papers published in reputable international scientific journals or from the findings of international panels of experts about the potential causes of breast (and prostate) cancer. Let me summarize what all this information means.

+ A rational explanation of cause and effect has been found now for many types of cancer, following Professor Richard Doll's breakthrough in the 1950s, which showed the link between smoking tobacco and lung cancer. For many types of cancer, we know that the disease is caused or triggered by something we do or are exposed to, including industrial chemicals and viral or bacterial infections. Some members of the exposed population may be more likely to be affected because of their genetic makeup, but many cancers for which there is now a well-established rational cause are related to lifestyle or environmental factors.
+ The incidence of breast cancer in some Western countries, and especially on the eastern seaboard of the United States, which includes many ethnic groups and hence a mixed gene pool, is similar to that of the incidence of lung cancer among heavy smokers. *This*

strongly suggests that something is causing the disease and that the cause relates to something that the higher socioeconomic groups in rich countries are doing.

+ Eastern communities have traditionally had exceptionally low rates of breast and prostate cancer (compared with Western countries). However, when Eastern people move to live in the West, their rates of breast and prostate cancer approach those of Western countries.

+ The rates of breast and prostate cancer also increase when Eastern people adopt a Western lifestyle in their own countries: in China the slang name for breast cancer translates as "Rich Woman's Disease." Typically Eastern diets have included most of the things eaten in the West, including meat such as pork, chicken, and duck (although in smaller quantities), but traditionally Eastern diets have *not* included dairy products.

+ The consumption of Western food, including dairy products such as milk, ice cream, and reprocessed dairy cow meat as in sausages and burgers, is increasing as countries like Japan embrace "development." This process of Westernization typically begins in urban centers. Breast and prostate cancer rates are increasing in these countries, and as we have seen from the data in Chapter 3, breast and prostate cancer rates in Eastern countries are significantly higher in urban than in rural areas.

+ Modern genetic research and molecular protein studies indicate that in the case of breast cancer the damage to the cell, which causes the wrong chain of protein signals to be relayed, leading to the uncontrolled growth that is cancer, is at a superficial level in the cell (between the receptors and intercellular fluid)—not deep inside the cell as is the case in some other types of cancers.

+ Only 5 to 10 percent of breast cancers are the result of inherited mutated (damaged) genes (BRCA-1 and BRCA-2), which are called tumor suppressor genes. These genes normally produce proteins to slow down cell growth. However, the disease does not always develop even in those carrying the mutated gene. This observation and the fact that they are tumor suppressor genes suggests that even where people have inherited mutated genes, their risk of cancer *can be reduced* if factors signaling the cell to produce too much or the wrong sorts of growth factors are removed.

+ Milk and the meat of dairy animals contain significant amounts of a growth factor called insulin-like growth factor-1, or IGF-1, and hormones such as prolactin.

+ The levels of IGF-1 in milk have probably increased due to selective stock breeding and the adoption of high-yielding species for dairying. Available estrogen levels may also have increased, because pregnant cows now continue to be milked.

+ The use of the genetically engineered hormone recombinant bovine growth hormone (rBGH), or bovine somatotropin (BST), to increase milk yield is associated with IGF-1 levels in milk at the highest part of the normal range.

+ IGF-1 and prolactin are known to promote the growth of breast and prostate cancer cells in laboratory cultures. This strongly suggests that they can do the same in humans, too, if they enter the bloodstream. Breast tissue has receptors for IGF-1, IGF-2, and prolactin.

+ Casein, the main milk protein, has been shown to protect growth hormones contained in milk from being broken down during digestion.

+ Modern methods of processing milk (including, for instance, homogenization) may further protect the cancer-promoting chemicals from breaking down in the gut, so that significant quantities are absorbed into the bloodstream. The direct effect of these chemicals on the digestive tract has been suggested by some scientists to cause colon cancer.

+ Research on humans shows that premenopausal women with high levels of circulating IGF-1 have a higher risk of breast cancer, and men with high levels of this circulating growth factor are at greater risk of suffering from prostate cancer than those with lower levels.

I RECOMMEND

Overall, I find the evidence of a connection between dairy product consumption and breast and prostate cancer compelling. It would, for example, explain the increase in breast and prostate cancer incidence with increasing age if, by consuming dairy products on a daily basis, we are exposing breast and prostate tissue, which should be turning off or turned off, to growth factors and hormones designed to cause the tissue to grow and proliferate. In the first version of this book, which was printed in the United Kingdom, I wrote:

> However, further research is needed to confirm the hypothesis. For example, studies are needed to show the extent to which those consuming dairy products, and certain types of meat prepared in different ways, have higher levels of free circulating IGF-1 in their blood than those consuming traditional Eastern diets. This should be carried out in experiments timed to follow consumption of suspect food types. Such research should be carried out by scientists working in independent organisations entirely free from commercial or political pressure. In the meantime, I recommend that all women who wish to prevent or treat breast cancer and all men who wish to prevent or treat prostate cancer *totally eliminate all forms of dairy produce from cows, sheep, goats or any animal milk from their diet.* The precautionary principle should be applied with the onus on the dairy industry to prove their product is safe.

Since I wrote that, research carried out at the Cancer Epidemiology Unit at Oxford University[77] and published in 2000 in the United Kingdom has shown that serum IGF-1 was 9 percent lower in 233 vegan men than in 226 meat-eaters (also thought to consume dairy products) and 237 ovo-lacto vegetarians. Remember that Chan and coworkers[78] found that men who subsequently developed prostate cancer had only 8 percent higher serum IGF-1 concentrations than men who remained healthy.

THE RISK WE RUN

I know that many people who read this book or hear about its suggestions will say that they have consumed dairy products all their lives with no ill effect—just as there are people who point out that they or someone they know has smoked two or three packs of cigarettes a day and lived to be 100. The problem is one of increasing risk to those in the population who, for genetic or other reasons, are more vulnerable. Risk is a difficult idea to explain. Many scientists who are specialists in risk (which is a concept based on probabilities) point out that no one would buy lottery tickets if they understood the subject, but human behavior is based more on personal experience and emotions than on mathematical concepts.

The best way of explaining cancer risk is perhaps the airplane analogy, which I use to try to persuade people to stop smoking. According to this example, you should think about how you would feel if you were going to fly in an airplane and you knew with certainty that one of every ten flights was going to crash. Would you fly? I don't think you would! Perhaps because they understand risk, very few scientists I know smoke.

I have never smoked, and knowing that I am vulnerable to breast cancer I will no longer eat any dairy products (including meat from animals used for dairying) in any form, at any time. I have lived without any dairy products whatsoever in my diet for almost seven years. Since I wrote that, a large cancer in my neck that was thought to be incurable shriveled and disappeared and has not returned. My previously brittle nails are now long and strong, my skin is in excellent condition, and I have no signs of osteoporosis. My hair is in excellent condition with very few gray hairs, and most people think I am much younger than my 55 years. I feel fitter and healthier than ever before.

I believe that I, and all those who have suffered from breast cancer but shared in my advice, have avoided death by dairy.

I have discovered recently that I am not the first person to say this. For example, Dr. R. M. Kradjian, M.D., Chief of the Breast Surgery Division of General Surgery at the Seton Medical Center, Daly City, California, has reached conclusions similar to my own. In his book *Save Yourself from Breast Cancer*,[79] and the "Milk Letter, a message to my patients,"[80] Dr. Kradjian strongly discourages all use of dairy products including nonfat milk, yogurt, and cheese. One of the facts he points out is that it is difficult to design a diet that is deficient in calcium when there are sufficient calories to meet daily needs. In addition to the links between dairy consumption and the diseases I have discussed, Dr. Kradjian also cites evidence of links with leukemia.

5.

The Plant Program—
The Food Factors

In this chapter I explain the seven dietary factors that can help you cut your risk of suffering from breast or prostate cancer.

First of all, let me say that The Plant Program *isn't* a diet. Diets, as many of us know from personal experience, generally don't work. Diets aren't much fun to follow, and sooner or later, we slide back to our old ways.

Instead, The Plant Program consists of seven Food Factors and five Lifestyle Factors, which together I have used to overcome advanced breast cancer and which I continue to follow to keep myself cancer-free against all the odds. The Plant Program not only helps to prevent and overcome breast and prostate cancer but is also protective against osteoporosis and other ills that are wrongly supposed to accompany a dairy-free diet. Together, these factors are quite easy to incorporate into your life: they should be seen as helping hands, not as severe dietary constraints.

The Plant Program is not a general anticancer diet like the Bristol and Gerson diets. As discussed earlier, cancers and their causes are different. The program that I describe here is targeted specifically at breast and prostate cancer and aims to eliminate or reduce chemicals in our food and from the environment that could disrupt our endocrine systems (the systems by which chemical messengers—especially hormones—regulate body function). The program is also designed to ensure that the body has available to it the chemicals, such as iodine and zinc, that it needs to maintain breast and prostate tissue in a healthy condition.

The main aims of the program are to:

+ Reduce the intake of hormones, including growth factors, from food and of man-made chemicals for which there is evidence or a suspicion of carcinogenicity, including endocrine-disrupting chemicals.

+ Increase the proportion of food containing substances that are protective against cancer.

+ Ensure that the body has adequate quantities of the key nutrients in a bioavailable form, so that at least a significant proportion can be absorbed by the body, especially nutrients such as zinc, iodine, and folic acid, which play a crucial role in cell division in the body (when the errors causing cancer are most likely to arise).

+ Reduce the amount of free radicals in the body that are capable of damaging DNA.

+ Give emphasis to food that is organically grown and as fresh as possible.

+ Eliminate or reduce to a minimum food that has been refined, tinned, preserved, or overcooked so that its content of fiber, vitamins, minerals, natural colors, or other natural constituents has been removed or reduced. (For example, molasses contains fluoride, which is protective against tooth decay, but in the refined white sugar prepared from molasses, fluoride and other nutrients have been removed, so we have to add fluoride to our toothpaste.) The aim is to eat whole food that has not been tampered with by the food processing industry and that does not contain chemical preservatives. Chemical preservatives and other additives are usually denoted in lists of ingredients on food labels by E numbers or chemical names. For further details see *Secret Ingredients* by Peter Cox and Peggy Brusseau (New York: Bantam, 1998).

+ Provide the nutrients to help your body withstand and recover from surgery, radiation therapy, and chemotherapy. The tips to help with radiation therapy described here are based on treatment methods developed to help astronauts withstand irradiation while in space. Many drugs, including those used in chemotherapy, destroy vitamins. Also, stress means you need more vitamins, and antibiotics can prevent them from being absorbed.

+ Provide maximum choice and variety so that healthy eating can be maintained without excessive dependence on any one type of food.

BASED ON GOOD SCIENCE

It is acknowledged by such authorities as the U.S. Food and Drug Administration and the British Department of Health as well as cancer specialists at Harvard University in the United States and Oxford University in Britain that diet accounts for at least 30 percent of all cancers. According to the Mayo Clinic in Rochester, Minnesota, individuals who eat five servings of fruit and vegetables a day (including cruciferous vegetables—that is, plants of the cabbage family whose four-petal flowers resemble a cross—such as bok choy, broccoli, brussels sprouts, cauliflower, cabbage, kale, kohlrabi, and watercress) cut their risk of cancer by half when compared with those consuming one serving or less. In Britain, official government advice now recommends that we eat at least five portions of fruit and vegetables a day, and following the pioneering work of Michael B. Sporn, Professor of Pharmacology and Medicine at Dartmouth Medical School, it is now widely acknowledged that plants contain many anticancer chemicals, the most important of which are described in the following pages.[1]

No intelligent doctor, therefore, should object to any of the scientifically based recommendations of The Plant Program. So why is it that when you mention using diet as part of your treatment for cancer, there is normally such a negative or, at best, lukewarm response from orthodox doctors?

I think there are several reasons. First, some people use such extreme diets that they become undernourished at a time when they need all their strength. Frequently this is because they have been to a type of alternative health practitioner who has recommended a diet typically eliminating red meat, wheat products, and processed food containing salt and sugar, along with tea, coffee, and alcohol. At the same time they are told to consume large quantities of fruit—often grapefruit—to "detoxify" the body, together with some vegetables, the list of which varies according to the practitioner. The diet recommended may be poorly balanced and not nutritious, with too few available nutrients. To make up for these deficiencies, synthetic vitamin and mineral supplements (sometimes the practitioner's own label marketed at excessive prices) are recommended. Sometimes the diets are developed by asking patients to hold or even think about a piece of food. Their muscle strength is then tested by pushing against the arm of the practitioner to determine their "food allergies." Some of my friends with a range of illnesses have ended up with the most ridiculous diets as a result. Often, when they have become undernourished or even more ill, a husband or family member has asked me to intervene. I have to say that I regard this method of developing a diet as complete mumbo jumbo—certainly I can see no scientific basis in it whatsoever.

There are other alternative "health practitioners" who use methods that are ill founded. For example, I remember talking to a homeopath I met at Charing Cross Hospital (she did not work there). She was visiting a patient with stomach cancer whom she was "treating" with ground-up granite. She was doing this on the basis that rates of stomach cancer are high in Wales where the rocks are granite. Hence, she argued, small quantities of ground-up granite would help the patient to ward off its effects in causing cancer. The homeopath was somewhat abashed when I pointed out to her that there is almost no granite in Wales and certainly not in the area where the rate of stomach cancer is high. I even brought a geologic map of Wales into the clinic to prove the point! I hope her patient's health was not made too much worse by her ministrations. I was also concerned to learn that some homeopaths prescribe preparations of radioactive salts such as radium bromide to prevent the side effects of radiation therapy. Even if these chemicals are highly diluted, the use of such preparations goes against all my scientific training, which seeks always to minimize exposure to radioactive substances.

But it's not only uninformed alternative health practitioners who sometimes give advice that is cause for concern. Several books on breast cancer have been published recently that also contain dubious advice. For example, one book implies that having more children at a younger age and breast-feeding them would protect against breast cancer. The suggestion that childbirth *protects* against breast cancer goes back to the observation that nuns in Italy suffered high levels of the disease. However, this observation doesn't prove that pregnancy and lactation can shield you from breast cancer, any more than celibacy might increase your risk. It is important to remember that many convents and monasteries housed very well-fed people: my speculation is that the nuns affected were consuming a rich diet containing lots of dairy products (and meat). In any case, I can find no evidence that statistical tests were carried out to see whether or not their rates of breast cancer were higher or lower than those of their host community. As discussed previously, modern statistical evidence suggests that being childless or postponing childbearing until later in life may increase risks *slightly*; but this could be just another index of women following a Western lifestyle and diet, since career women in particular tend to delay childbearing.

The strongest evidence on the cause of breast and prostate cancer suggests that it is linked to our consumption of dairy food—which is not designed for adult humans and which we have not evolved to eat, especially now that it is produced by intensive industrialized methods. Also, a number of pollutants, including endocrine-disrupting chemicals from the environment—many of which are fat-soluble and accumulate up the food chain—become particularly concentrated in milk. Growing population pressure is one of the drivers of the industrialization of agriculture and chemical pollution. Hence, increasing pregnancy rates would exacerbate, not alleviate, the burden of breast and prostate cancer for society as a whole.

Nor do I think that factors such as using mobile phones or deodorants or wearing incorrectly fitting bras cause breast cancer. Breast cancer was a feature of Western societies long before these relatively modern inventions. Clearly we should not wear bras that are too small to the extent that they stop circulation, but do women, especially middle-class women, really go around wearing such tight bras? The idea that we should all buy new bras may be good for bra sales, but I suggest that it has little to do with breast cancer. Mobile phones may be implicated in causing problems with the head and brain, although existing research is inconclusive, but breast cancer rates had been rising for a long time before the use of mobile phones. In one recent article in the Canadian press, a group of women made the case for breast cancer being caused by their working in an office equipped with computers and other electronic equipment. The main advocate of this idea is pictured drinking a large milkshake! In the case of the contraceptive pill, young women taking it do not have an appreciably increased risk of breast cancer. Any small increase in relative risk disappears ten years after they stop using it. There is, however, evidence of increased incidence of breast cancer in women who have used the pill until their early 40s.[2]

Many anti-breast-cancer diets that appear in magazines seem to have no scientific basis or even logic. For example, in a magazine published recently by a health food shop, the same article that promotes the use of soy as part of an anti-breast-cancer diet recommends *against* chickpeas and lentils. Did the author not know that these foods are all legumes and contain similar isoflavone chemicals? Moreover, the same author includes soy, oat, and rice milk under the heading of dairy products along with goats' milk! A national newspaper recently serialized an anti-breast-cancer diet book that claimed that parsnips, potatoes, broad beans, pumpkins, honey, watermelon, pineapple, couscous, and muesli (all of which I believe to be good foods and of which I eat masses) increase the risk of breast cancer because they stimulate "excess insulin" production. These foods were lumped together with processed foods such as commercial refined breakfast cereals, chocolate bars, and jelly beans! This is certainly advice I shall choose to ignore. Yet another recent breast cancer diet book enthusiastically recommended consuming live yogurt as a chemopreventive food—again with no scientific basis. A recent article on bowel cancer in a magazine linked to several cancer charities advocated consuming "high-calcium foods, i.e., dairy products (choose low-fat cheese and semiskimmed milk), which are thought to help protect you." Calcium has been shown to be a factor in bowel cancer, but in the context of malnutrition.[3] And of course, it can be obtained from sources much healthier than dairy (see p. 124). No wonder people are confused about healthy eating.

Most other recent anticancer diets are based on the principles first set out in the Max Gerson diet published in 1953. Dr. Gerson's basic precept was that cancer is a symptom of a diseased body in which the organs— especially the liver—are out of balance. So he reasoned that most animal products, salt, and caffeine should be banned to take the pressure off the liver and immune system, and the body should be detoxified and rebalanced using organic fruit and vegetables in order to cure cancer. In his book entitled *A Cancer Therapy*, the following substances are forbidden:

tobacco, salt, sharp spices, tea, coffee, cocoa, chocolate, alcohol, refined sugar, refined flour, candies, ice cream, cream, cake, nuts, mushrooms, all soy products, pickles, pineapples, berries, avocados, cucumbers, water (you are supposed to drink only fresh juices), canned, preserved, or sulfured food, smoked or salted vegetables, dehydrated or bottled juices, all fats, oils, salt substitutes, and all sources of fluoride. Butter, cheese, fish, meat, eggs, and milk were forbidden during initial treatment, although, confusingly, cottage cheese, buttermilk, and yogurt are mentioned in the specific section on cancer therapy and are included in the sample menus. Unfortunately, Gerson also recommended raw calves' liver juice as a source of nutrients (not recommended in the post-BSE era) and the use of coffee and castor oil enemas. Gerson published his diet well before the present level of industrialization of agriculture, but he foresaw the dangers of degrading our environment, particularly of depleting soils of nutrients and polluting them with chemicals.

Gerson's regimen as a treatment for cancer is outlawed in most American states, which his daughter Charlotte blames on "the lucrative drug industry."[4] The Gerson method is rigorous, lengthy, and time-consuming, demands absolute commitment, and includes preparing and immediately drinking fresh organic juices every hour (twelve times a day). Many British doctors are skeptical about the value of the Gerson method. Dr. Slavin of Saint Bartholomew's Hospital, London, is quoted in *The* (London) *Times*, 2 November 1999 as saying, "I would like to say I had seen improvement in even one patient I know of who has taken the therapy, but I have not." Nevertheless, many people do attest to the Gerson method having worked for them, although such cases are generally dismissed by doctors as "anecdotal."

The Gerson diet was my starting point, but I have made many modifications. I removed some "allowed foods" and encourage the consumption of some "forbidden foods" such as soy products and berries. My diet is based on modern scientific research findings and is specific for breast and prostate cancer. I have also eliminated suggestions for which I can find no scientific basis, especially those that make the diet unnecessarily difficult to follow and keep to. The Bristol diet developed by Dr. Alec Forbes is based on principles similar to those of the Gerson diet, to which Dr. Forbes refers, but there are variations in the list of good and bad foods. As indicated earlier (see pp. 38–39), following the Bristol diet did not help me.

One of the main reasons many Western doctors find it difficult to accept diet as part of cancer treatment is that they are trained to administer chemicals, which are pure substances in measurable doses with a defined (stoichiometric) formula. The chemicals have usually been tested on cultures, animals, and finally humans using statistically designed studies. We have all seen old movies, especially Westerns, where some charlatan or quack is peddling a cure for something that is just a way of making money. Modern clinical medicine is designed to prevent this type of thing from happening. Nevertheless, many Western doctors could be given better training in the nutritional and environmental factors that can promote disease. In the case of breast and prostate cancer, such an understanding is essential if diets are to be used in the same way as they are in treating coronary heart disease or diabetes, for example. I believe that the program described here provides a sound basis to help doctors and other health professionals help their patients. I used it to recover from what would otherwise have been terminal breast cancer and observed on a day-to-day basis the effect it had on a large visible cancer in my neck. The program also helped prevent any hair loss during chemotherapy. I have lived on the program for almost seven years with no sign of undernourishment despite what many people would describe as a punishing work schedule with lots of responsibility, long hours of work, and international travel. Most people think I look very healthy and that I am much younger than my 55 years. I have not had a day's serious illness since my treatment for cancer ended. Indeed, many irritating problems that had troubled me for years, such as cold sores, throat infections, thrush, candida, brittle nails, which often had infections around their base, and recurrent cystitis, have all cleared up. Also, since I adopted The Plant Program, my rate of tooth decay has decreased markedly. I have given the diet to sixty-three women, all of whom remain cancer-free. These women range from the 70-year-old mother of a Canadian friend, with advanced breast cancer that had spread to her bones, to a young Englishwoman whose breast cancer was diagnosed when she was breast-feeding her first baby. The five women who refused to use it or "cheated" have all sadly had recurrences or have died.

Undoubtedly, the best anticancer diet would be completely vegan (strictly vegetarian, with no meat or dairy products). I was living on a completely vegan diet at the time my cancer disappeared and for about eight months afterward. If you can become a vegan, so much the better, but you must ensure that you don't become deficient in essential nutrients such as zinc and selenium and vitamins such as D and B_{12}. However, do not confuse being vegan with becoming a vegetarian. Vegetarians sometimes consume far more dairy products (to replace meat) than other members of society, and some processed, prepackaged vegetarian foods can have particularly high contents of dairy products. If you want to reduce your risk of breast (or prostate) cancer, become a vegan *but on no account become a dairy-eating vegetarian*. If any anticancer diet includes any dairy products of any kind, ignore it.

For a long time many middle-class women I know have been substituting cottage cheese and yogurt for red meat in their diet, partly influenced by health and lifestyle magazines and partly by animal rights activists such as Linda McCartney, who recently died of breast cancer. For many busy women, eating yogurt or cheese is simpler and therefore less time-consuming than creating balanced vegan meals to reduce meat consumption, and I suspect that an overall increase in dairy consumption has been the result.

Many women have been persuaded that they need to consume dairy products for the calcium they contain—especially to ward off osteoporosis, a skeletal disorder of progressive bone mass loss and demineralization causing increased risk of fracture. Milk and milk products do indeed contain significant amounts of calcium, but calcium is most definitely not synonymous with dairy. In any case, ingesting large quantities of calcium does not, in itself, seem to eliminate bone loss:

+ A 1987 Mayo Clinic study, which examined dietary calcium intake and actual rates of bone loss in women, determined that "these data do not support the hypothesis that insufficient dietary calcium is a major cause of bone loss in women."[5]
+ Many populations with high intakes of calcium also have high rates of osteoporosis.[6]
+ The Inuit, for example, consume twice the amount of calcium found in the average Western diet (about 2,000 mg daily). This

does not prevent them from suffering from high rates of osteoporosis, and it has been estimated that compared with U.S. Caucasians, the Inuit have an average of 10 to 15 percent less bone mass. This is probably due to the Inuit's considerable intake of protein (250 to 400 grams daily) from fish, whale, and walrus.[7]

+ On the other hand, Bantus living in Africa on low-calcium (400 mg daily) and low-protein vegetable diets (47 grams daily) are essentially free of osteoporosis.[8]

The World Health Organization confirms that countries with relatively low intakes of calcium do not have an increased incidence of osteoporosis. Indeed, they note the suggestion that dietary calcium levels not too different from those proposed to prevent osteoporosis can cause a number of adverse biological effects.[9] The British government's own nutritional advisory panel confirms this paradox: "Several populations of the world consume calcium at levels lower than the current RDA for the UK yet show no evidence of adverse effects."[10] Careful scientific studies into calcium absorption (using radioactive labeling techniques) have shown that only 18 to 36 percent of the calcium in milk is taken up by the body.[11] This is taken into account by the authorities responsible for setting recommended nutrient intakes, who generally assume that something in the range of 20 to 40 percent of the diet's calcium content is actually absorbed, and therefore build a "safety factor" for this into their figures.

Some nutrition textbooks, perhaps without always checking to see if the effect is more theoretical than real, argue that certain plants contain chemicals that bind with calcium in the gut so that only a small proportion is absorbed. The American Dietetic Association comments on this question: "Calcium absorption appears to be inhibited by such plant constituents as phytic acid, oxalic acid, and fiber, but this effect may not be significant. Calcium deficiency in vegetarians is rare and there is little evidence to show that low intakes of calcium give rise to major health problems among the vegetarian population."[12] Dr. Neal Barnard, president of the Physicians Committee for Responsible Medicine, summarizes the evidence thus: "The amount of calcium in your bones is very carefully regulated by hormones. Increasing your calcium intake does not fool those hormones into building more bone, any more than delivering an extra

TABLE 3: PROPOSED CALCIUM INTAKE REQUIREMENT FOR WOMEN

AGE	MG
Normal adult	800
Adolescent growth	1,100
Pregnancy	1,000
Lactation	1,200
Elderly with HRT	1,000
Elderly without HRT	1,500

load of bricks will make a construction crew build a larger building. . . . For the vast majority of people, the answer is not boosting your calcium intake, but rather, limiting calcium loss."[13]

The wisdom of these words contrasts with the prevailing recommendations of other authorities. Currently, the adult recommended daily intake for calcium is about 700 mg a day. Yet a U.S. experts' conference on osteoporosis put the recommended level as high as 1,500 mg per day for women,[14] and a British symposium on osteoporosis has proposed the intakes for women shown in Table 4.

At the upper level, an intake of 1,500 mg of calcium a day would have to be supplied by nearly half a pound of hard cheese, four cartons of yogurt, or five cups of milk!

Many plants contain large quantities of calcium. Good nondairy sources of calcium are dark green leafy vegetables (such as kale, collards, turnip greens, and broccoli). One study shows that 27 percent of the calcium in watercress can be absorbed. Another study has demonstrated that calcium absorbability is actually higher for kale than for milk, and concludes: "greens such as kale can be considered to be at least as good as milk in terms of their calcium absorbability."[15] Other calcium-rich vegetables include artichokes, cabbage, carrots, celery, celery root, chickpeas, Chinese cabbage, chives, watercress, dandelion leaves, fennel, French beans, horseradish, leeks, onions, parsley, parsnips, and spinach, although the exact quantities they contain vary. The fruits that are richest in calcium include rosehips, raspberries, oranges, kiwi, figs, blackcurrants, and blackberries. Other good sources are almonds, tofu, soy flour, string beans, oatmeal and whole wheat flour, pumpkin, sesame, and sunflower seeds, seaweed, and dried fruit. Using soy products provides calcium and magnesium together with iron and in a better balance than milk. Moreover, some soy milk has calcium added to it. Hummus (made from chickpeas and sesame) is also a rich source of calcium. Some beers also contain concentrations of calcium—many breweries were set up in areas where the level of gypsum, the most soluble bioavailable form of mineral calcium, is naturally high in the water used for brewing. Other beers are rich in magnesium and phosphorus.

Of equal importance is the need to reduce calcium loss from your body. Here are some points to remember:

+ A diet high in animal-based proteins increases the amount of acid in the body. This triggers a buffering mechanism, which releases stored calcium from the bones. The body would normally reabsorb the calcium released, but the animal protein inhibits the parathyroid function that controls this reabsorption. The body then excretes the calcium, causing bone loss. One researcher who put this theory to the test concluded: "This study suggests that a diet higher in vegetable protein might actually be somewhat protective against osteoporosis."[16]

+ Reduce caffeine consumption. A study of women aged 36 to 45 found that those who drank two cups of coffee a day suffered a net calcium loss of 22 mg daily. Reducing this to one cup daily reduced the loss to just 6 mg daily.[17]

+ Reduce alcohol consumption. Alcohol speeds bone loss because it interferes with the way your body absorbs calcium. When you drink, drink mainly beer, as many beers contain high levels of calcium and have a lower alcohol content than most alcoholic drinks.

+ Get some sun. Sunlight reacts with dehydrocholesterol in your skin to produce vitamin D, which is essential to the proper absorption of calcium, and a deficiency will cause you to lose bone mass.

+ Magnesium works with other vitamins and minerals, including calcium, to promote bone growth and the healthy functioning of nerves and muscle tissue. A deficiency of magnesium can affect the manufacture of vitamin D, so it is important in preventing osteoporosis. Magnesium is a constituent of chlorophyll and so is abundant in green vegetables. Other excellent sources are whole grains, wheat germ, molasses, seeds and nuts, apples, and figs.

+ The trace mineral boron helps to prevent calcium loss and is thought to help in the manufacture of vitamin D in the body. Foods naturally rich in boron are easily obtained and include most fruits, particularly apples, berries, grapes, pears, prunes, dates, raisins, tomatoes, almonds, peanuts, and hazelnuts.

+ Get some exercise. Weight-bearing exercise is important in building and maintaining bones.

+ Above all, increase your intake of phytoestrogens and phytoprogesterones by following the program described below.

Below are the seven Food Factors that, together with the five Lifestyle Factors discussed in Chapter 6, comprise The Plant Program. If you are using The Plant Program to prevent cancer, I suggest that you incorporate the factors into your life at your own pace, proceeding from one to the next as you feel ready and able to do so. If you have active cancer, I suggest that you try to make all the adjustments as quickly as possible. Before you begin, it is worth making the general point that adding good foods that contain anticancer agents to a diet that continues to include other potentially harmful components will not, in my experience, help. For this reason, and as explained fully under Food Factor 2 (see p. 141), I recommend that, as much as possible, all the foodstuffs you consume be organically produced.

FOOD FACTOR 1: FULL OF BEANS

One of the first and most essential things you can do to reduce your risk of breast cancer and probably prostate cancer is to substitute soy products for dairy products (whether from cows, sheep, goats, or other animal species) in your diet. Replace animal milk with soy, rice, oat, or coconut milk; replace cheese with tofu; and eat soy ice cream (or water ices or sorbets) instead of dairy ice cream. There are no half measures here, and as discussed previously, using skim milk or low-fat yogurt will not help to reduce your risk of breast cancer or increase your ability to recover from the disease, because some of the most likely cancer-causing agents in diary products are proteins, not fats.* Indeed, recent research suggests that any *protective* factors against breast cancer contained in milk are likely to be in the fat, not the protein. Conjugated linoleic acid (CLA), which is created by bacteria in the stomachs of cattle and which is found in milk fat, has been suggested to inhibit the growth of cancer. Hence removing fat from milk could make the risk of cancer from consuming dairy products *worse* in some respects. Work at the University of Utah is aimed at increasing the CLA levels of milk, but, of course, it will not increase the CLA content of skim milk. However, before you decide to have cream or butter, bear in mind that man-made organochlorines, some of which are implicated in breast cancer (see Chapter 6), are mainly concentrated in the fat.

All dairy products should be avoided and replaced by soy products. By making this group of changes to your diet, you will immediately and dramatically reduce your body's exposure to a powerful cocktail of hormones shown in experiment after experiment to promote breast and prostate cancer cell growth in cultures and/or experimental animals. You will also be reducing your exposure to antibiotic residues and other powerful biologically active chemicals (including man-made endocrine-disrupting chemicals, which can become particularly concentrated in milk—see Chapter 6). You will be reducing your cholesterol and triglyceride intake with great benefits for your heart and circulatory system, thereby helping to deliver anticancer agents derived from plants (see Food Factor 2) to the site of any cancer tumor faster and more effectively. And you will reduce the possibility of developing thrombosis. Patients undergoing chemotherapy for breast cancer are especially susceptible to this. For example, the risk of thrombosis increased fivefold in a group receiving cyclophos-

---

*Interestingly, an amino acid in milk, meat, and some vegetables called methionine is increasingly being implicated in coronary heart disease.[18] Its metabolism in the absence of adequate folates (which are high in vegetables but low in dairy products) and vitamins B_6 and B_{12} produces high levels of a chemical called homocysteine, which is thought to be a determinant of cardiovascular disease. It has been suggested that most Americans ingesting the standard diet have high levels of circulating homocysteine.

phamide methotrexate and 5-fluorouracil, precisely the treatment I was given.[19]

Recent dietary studies into the effects of exchanging soy for animal products indicate a reduction in cholesterol levels of more than 20 percent. Moreover, it is the levels of the "bad" cholesterol—low-density lipoproteins, or LDLs—that are reduced. However, simply adding soy to a typical Western diet may not be sufficient to counteract high plasma cholesterol and platelet aggregation.[20] You must replace—not supplement—dairy with soy products to achieve the benefits. Remember that soy also contains plant estrogens that protect the breast in the same way that tamoxifen does, and one of the plant estrogens—genistein—seems to prevent cancer through multiple mechanisms: not only is it phytoestrogenic, it is anti-angiogenic, too, meaning that it actually prevents tumors from developing their own blood supply.[21] It is also a powerful antioxidant, increasing the activities of protective antioxidative enzymes in various organs, with an important role in the removal of free radicals, and, in particular, oxygen radicals, which have been particularly implicated in cancer. The vast majority of experimental studies into soy and cancer have shown that soybeans and soy products prevent the growth of a range of cancer cells.[22]

There is only one problem with buying soy now: it has often been genetically modified. One of the reasons this has been done is so that it can withstand being treated with pesticides and herbicides to destroy insects and weeds. So read labels carefully and buy only organically grown soy.

The soybean is one of the most nutritious vegetables known. It is said that the soybean was a gift to all generations of mankind from the sages and wise rulers of China. When the very first specimens of the soybean reached the West, at the end of the eighteenth century, their arrival coincided with the dawn of the Industrial Revolution. So it was the industrial uses of the soybean that captivated the entrepreneurial minds of those who came to inspect the first specimens grown in London's Royal Botanic Gardens. Consequently, the first commercial use for the soybean was as a source of oil to be used in the manufacture of soap, and the remains of the bean, after the oil had been extracted, were fed to cattle. This pattern of usage, so different from that in Asia, is at last beginning to change as more and more people appreciate the extraordinary health-giving properties of soy.

The soybean is an environmentally friendly crop, too. One acre of land cultivated by conventional Western agricultural practices will feed an average adult for 77 days if it is used to raise beef. This may seem impressive, until you learn that the same acre can feed an adult for 527 days when it is devoted to growing wheat. However, if soybeans are grown on the same land, then it will yield enough protein to feed a person for over six years! This phenomenal productivity is caused in part by the ability of the soybean, which is a legume, to fix atmospheric nitrogen into the soil through the action of bacteria on its roots. The protein content of the bean when harvested is about 40 percent, which rises to 50 percent after it has been processed. Soy also contains a full range of proteins, whereas other plant foods contain only some. Hence vegans depend on combining cereals and the edible seeds of legumes to obtain the full range of twenty amino acids necessary for good nutrition. The traditional Jamaican dish of rice and peas, which I eat a lot when I work there, is a good example. It is delicious.

Most of us are familiar with soy milk, which can be purchased from all supermarkets. However, that's just the tip of the iceberg: there are many other traditional soy products, which you will enjoy discovering and experimenting with. Let me introduce you to some of them.

Tofu

Tofu, or *fromage de soja* ("soy cheese") as it is known in France, is made from soybeans (you can make it yourself at home quite easily). It has a higher percentage of protein than any other natural food in existence, is very low in saturated fats, and is entirely cholesterol-free; at the same time it is inexpensive. It has been a staple food for millions of people in Asia for over 4,000 years. Tofu is very good for everyone, from very young children to the elderly, because it is so full of good nutrients, is so low in bad nutrients, and can be so easily digested. In their book *New Tofu Recipes,* Christopher and Jean Conil suggest that pured carrots and leeks with tofu can be used as a nutritious, easily digested food for babies and invalids. Also, for those short of time, tofu requires no lengthy cooking and can be simply stir-fried or simmered in soup. It is made by precipitating soy milk, normally using calcium or magnesium sulphates, so it is also high in some of the most bioavailable forms of calcium or magnesium. In their classic treatise on the subject, William Shurtleff and Akiko Aoyagi explain its revered status:

> Along with rice, wheat, barley and millet, soy beans were included among China's venerated *nuku* or five sacred grains, as early as the beginning of the Christian era . . . [and] the sense of the sacredness of soya bean foods is still alive in Japan today; here the words tofu, miso and shoyu are commonly preceded in everyday speech by the honorific prefix "O." Rather than saying tofu, most people say "O—tofu," meaning honourable tofu. Today, the soya bean has become the king of the Japanese kitchen. Indeed, the arrival of tofu, miso and shoyu in Japan initiated a revolution in the national cuisine. Now when Japanese connoisseurs speak of these foods, they use many of the same terms we employ when evaluating cheeses or wines; traditional tofu masters often say that the consummation of their art is but to evoke the fine flavours latent in the soya bean. And when the new crop of soya beans arrives at tofu shops late each autumn, ardent devotees sample the first tofu with the discrimination and relish of French vintners.[23]

In fact the Chinese emperor Shang Nung made the soy plant one of the five holy cultivated sources of protein in his celestial empire in 2838 B.C.

Commercially, tofu is available in either "silken" form (suitable for making low-fat, high-protein dressings and sauces) or firm, which can be used in an infinite number of ways: scrambled, marinated, smoked, barbecued, crumbled into salads, in burgers, sandwiches, and soups, or even in a dessert. Start to use it, and you'll be dazzled by its potential! Tofu may not taste good to you on its own, but as described in the Conils' *New Tofu Recipes,* "It has magical properties of absorbing almost any flavour or colour and so can be introduced in a wide range of dishes." There are many ways to flavor tofu. I usually use a base or marinade of miso, garlic, ginger, and onion for savory dishes. Tofu also works well with onion and celery and is ideal as a replacement for dairy cream or milk in many potato dishes. It can also be liquidized with a wide range of fresh or dried fruit previously soaked in juice to which honey has been added to make delicious sweets and desserts, to replace yogurt or ice cream, for example.

Tempeh

Tempeh (pronounced tem-pay) is a fermented soybean product, made in the traditional manner for centuries throughout Indonesia where it is a basic food for millions of people. You can buy it in every health food shop and a growing number of supermarkets. Like cheese, yogurt, and ginger beer, it is made with a cultured "starter." It is highly digestible, smells like fresh mushrooms, and tastes remarkably similar to chicken or veal outlets. Since the protein in tempeh is partially broken down during fermentation (the mold is called rhizopusoligosporus), it is a particularly suitable food for young children and older people. Tempeh is typically sold in six-inch squares that are approximately one inch thick. The easiest way to serve it is to cut the square in half diagonally, and then cut each half into three thinner, wedge-shaped slices. These should then be panfried until crisp and golden brown on both sides, and then served with rice and a selection of vegetables. Shoyu or tamari sprinkled over the top will give it a little extra flavoring; alternatively, mix with lemon juice for a truly sensational marinade.

Miso

Miso is a fermented mixture of soybeans and some other cereal grain, such as rice or barley, and is pastelike in appearance and texture. It is an important component of Eastern-based macrobiotic diets. It has subtle, aromatic flavors and comes in many different colors, including orange, brown, and yellow. It is one of the staples of every Japanese and Chinese kitchen. It is made by inoculating the basic ingredients with a mold (*koji*) and is then aged in cedarwood kegs for at least one year. It is most commonly used as an ingredient in soups, sauces, dressings, spreads, casseroles, and other vegetable dishes. The miso industry is among the largest food industries in Japan today, and synthetic misos, which would include various colorings and additives, are quite widely available. Buy only traditionally made miso, since not only is it free of additives, but the complex fermentation process produces a wealth of substances such as enzymes and beneficial bacteria that have a positive effect upon human health. Also buy only good reputable brands of miso because fermentation in unhygienic conditions can cause high concentrations of the microorganisms thought to be responsible for stomach cancer. I buy miso only in waxed cartons, never in plastic (see p. 201). The valuable mineral nutrients in miso and other cereals are far more accessible to the body after fermentation than those in raw cereals. (The banning of fermentation of cereals by well-meaning missionaries trying to prevent alcohol consumption is one of the contributors to malnutrition in grain-based societies in Africa today.) In Japan, miso is commonly respected as a food that is also a medicine. The various types of miso include:

+ Hacho miso—soybean miso, the heartiest and thickest of all, having a rich, almost chocolate-like flavor
+ Mugi miso—barley miso, made with a combination of soybeans and barley, a mellow-tasting miso whose color can range from almost white through yellow to red
+ Kome miso—rice miso, made from a combination of soybeans, rice, and sea salt, the most commonly consumed in Japan, with a light and almost sweet taste

A simple miso soup can be made by lightly sautéing a selection of sliced vegetables (onions, leeks, turnips, potatoes) in a small amount of oil, then adding water and slowly simmering the vegetables for about half an hour. Finally, turn off the heat and add a good dollop of miso to flavor. Add a strip of kombu or wakame seaweed before serving. On no account should the soup be boiled with the miso in it, because this will destroy many of the beneficial, health-giving substances including vitamins that live miso contains, while boiling the seaweed would drive off the iodine.

Soy Sauce

Soy sauce is an ancient and traditional Japanese seasoning that has achieved prominence and acceptance the world over. It is a dark, rich sauce with a savory, salty taste as well as a deep, mellowing background flavor. Very little is required within a dish or serving. There are three types:

The first is a commercial, accelerated-production type that is widely available and usually sold as soy sauce. It is made by speeding the process of fermentation using chemical additives. It usually contains colorings and preservatives as well. I do not recommend it.

The second is called *shoyu* and is made by fermenting wheat and soybeans together for at least three years. During this time the flavor develops, making it a delicious addition to most savory meals. The amino acids present in the ferment aid digestion. It is easy to find in health food, macrobiotic, or Japanese grocery shops.

The third is *tamari,* which is made by fermenting just soybeans and salt over a long period of time, between two and three years. It is less widely available than shoyu because traditionally much less of it is made. It is not used so often in cooking or as a table condiment as shoyu because its flavor is much stronger.

Both shoyu and tamari are fermented with *koji,* a mold that grows at the temperature of the human body and develops enzymes helpful in the digestion of proteins and starches, similar to those found in human saliva.

Natto

Though less readily available than tempeh at the moment, natto can generally be found in Chinese or Japanese grocery stores. Like tempeh, it is made by fermenting soybeans, but in this case, for less than 24 hours. It has an intriguing gossamer-like quality and is one of the most unusual foods you will ever eat. The fermentation process makes the high-quality protein of the soybeans particularly easy to digest. Serve natto in a small bowl beside a serving of freshly steamed rice, stir-fried vegetables, and your favorite dipping sauce.

From Dairy to Soy

Good soy and tofu products are widely available not only in specialist health food shops but also in supermarkets, so there is no difficulty in buying them. Since there are so many different types and flavors, it is worth experimenting until you find the flavors you enjoy. As described above, I also use tofu to make delicious desserts and ice cream or yogurt substitutes based on whisking or liquidizing tofu with fruit and honey. Your brain will adapt to the change in taste quickly and you will soon find you do not want to go back to dairy products. Even the smell of milk is nauseating to me now—it smells of cows' udders! It reminds me of when I gave up taking sugar in tea. Before I did it, I thought the tea would taste horrible without sugar, but within a week of giving it up I found that tea with sugar tasted disgusting, and tea with sugar and milk: Ugh!

So what about yogurt and all those healthy lactobacillus acidophilus bacteria it contains that are so good for us? There is evidence that taking these bacteria increases immunity, prevents infections, and increases vitamin production. Actually, giving up dairy products doesn't mean that you have to sacrifice acidophilus, because it is easy to buy capsules of the bacteria and put them in soy milk or other cold drinks. Hence you have the health benefits of the bacteria without the risk that consuming dairy products carries. Moreover, following The Plant Program will favor the growth and survival of these helpful bacteria in the digestive tract.

It is also worth remembering that soy contains phytoestrogens and steroids that are progestogenic and can prevent menopausal symptoms. I carry a small jar of dried soy (WySoy) or a small soy milkshake with me everywhere I go—otherwise within a few hours of not taking it I have appalling hot flashes. I have helped many friends with their menopausal problems by persuading them to drink soy milk, and they are all amazed to find out how easy it is to eliminate hot flashes within days.

If you do only one thing to cut your risk of breast cancer (and I believe also prostate cancer), please make the change from dairy to soy products. Remember that soy products reduce breast cancer in laboratory experiments, while milk and the growth factors and other hormones it contains have been shown in experiment after experiment to promote the growth of breast and prostate cancer cells. Of the people who have followed my program, only those who have "cheated" on this aspect have ever had a return of breast cancer. When I asked one of my friends—who has recently had to have her second breast removed and now faces six months of chemotherapy—if she had kept to my diet (because if it does not work, I do not want to give people false hope), she said, "Well, I just couldn't resist cheese, and I am sure yogurt is good for you—everyone says it is."

There is one concern about eating food full of phytoestrogen that some men have expressed to me: that is that eating the phytoestrogens in soy will feminize them. Despite exhaustive studies, there is no evidence of this.[24] Moreover, a lack of male potency and reproductive capacity does not appear to have been a problem in China or other Eastern countries over the many centuries they have used soy. Rather the reverse.

MAKING THE BREAK:
How to Put More Beans into Your Life

If You Used to Do This . . .	Now Do This!
Take cows' milk in your tea or coffee	Use soy milk in tea, straight from the carton. In coffee, heat the soy milk first to avoid curdling. Avoid dry "creamers" without first reading their labels: many contain dairy milk proteins and/or fats.
Put cows' milk on your breakfast cereal	Use your favorite soy, rice, oat, or coconut milk, or pour fresh fruit juice over your cereal instead.
Tuck into a bowl of ice cream	Enjoy high-quality sorbets or water ices. Or try one of the growing range of soy ice creams now on the market.
Douse your desserts in cream or custard	Most supermarkets sell small cartons of a brand of soy "cream." To make your own, whisk soft plain tofu

If You Used to Do This . . .	Now Do This!
	with a little honey or malt extract for a thick, rich topping. One of the oldest brands of custard powder is dairy-free! Simply prepare it using soy milk instead of dairy. Or try one of the custardlike soy desserts now widely available.
Drink glasses of milk or milkshakes	Many producers offer a range of flavored or naturally sweetened soy, rice, oat, or coconut milks in various carton sizes. Or make your own ultrathick shake at home. See the recipes below.
Use dollops of butter in cooking or on bread or vegetables	Use organic first- and cold-pressed extra-virgin olive oil in cooking. Try herb-flavored olive oil drizzled over toast or baked potatoes, and lift your sandwiches with a spread such as tahini (sesame seed paste) to take the place of butter and to enhance your nutrient intake.
Eat masses of hard, soft, or cottage cheese	Several brands of dairy-free hard "cheeses" are currently available in health food shops, and these may be used in cookery as well as simply grated or sliced. Double-check the label to ensure the product is free from casein, lactose, and other "hidden" dairy ingredients. Soft soy "cheeses" abound—available as tofu dips, spreads, or pâtés, for instance. My favorite option is either tofu (smoked, marinated, braised, or plain) or hummus. I know it's not soy, but it has similar benefits.

If You Used to Do This . . .	Now Do This!
Dive into a daily dose of yogurt	Soy yogurt is widely available in plain and fruit flavors and in a variety of carton sizes.
Eat dairy (made from cow) meat products such as burgers, sausages, luncheon meats, pâtés, and pastes	A huge variety of products are now widely available to replace meat in all its guises. Look for these products in the dry mix, canned, frozen, or refrigerated food sections of your health food shop or supermarket. Although some of these products are based on nuts, most are based on soy (i.e., various tofus, tempeh, and texturized vegetable protein [TVP]) in ground or chunk form and in various savory flavors.
Cook with dairy products	Soy milk or cream readily substitutes for dairy milk in recipes as varied as béchamel sauce, creamed soups, rice pudding, and quiche. Most recipes calling for butter succeed as well with olive oil or Granose soy spread. The meat replacements mentioned above serve well in traditional recipes, as do the cheese substitutes.

Here are some sensational recipes by my friend Peggy Brusseau, which are quick, easy, and very tasty! Use them to effortlessly boost your intake of the soybean.

Chili without Carne

This dish was originally made with meat that was heavily spiced with chili peppers. The flavor, texture, and aroma of this meatless version are authentic and irresistible. Aim for a level of spiciness at the borders of your tolerance, and cook until the sauce has the consistency of ragout: thick and gloopy.

Serves 4
Preparation time 45 minutes

1 tbsp olive oil
5 cloves garlic, finely chopped
2 medium onions, thinly sliced
½–1 tsp chili powder
4 oz TVP ground
1 pint water
5 oz tomato puree
14 oz canned tomatoes or 6 medium tomatoes, chopped
1 whole chili pepper, to taste (optional)
1 lb cooked red kidney beans (optional)
2 tsp soy sauce
1 tbsp vinegar

Heat the oil in a saucepan and sauté the garlic and onion until clear and tender. Add the chili powder and sauté for a further 1 minute. Stir the TVP into the sauté to absorb all the oil and juices, then add the water, tomato puree, and chopped tomatoes. Stir well and reduce the heat to medium. Add the chili and/or red beans at this point and add a little more water if necessary to ensure the right consistency. Cover the pan, reduce the heat, and let simmer about 20 minutes. Add the soy sauce and vinegar about 5 minutes before serving. Serve hot in small bowls with a plate of fresh tortillas nearby and, if you're really keen, a small dish of fresh hot chilies!

If you like milkshakes, try—

Banana Shake

Serves 4
Preparation time 10 minutes

2 pints cold soy milk
4 very ripe bananas, peeled
2 oz ground almonds
½ tsp ground nutmeg

Place all the ingredients (or half at a time) in a blender and whisk to a thick, frothy consistency. Pour into chilled glasses and serve immediately with a garnish of flaked almonds or a single banana chip floating on the surface.

How about a stir-fry? Try—

Tofu Sukiyaki

Serves 4
Preparation time 45 minutes

4 oz ramen noodles
1 pint water
2 medium carrots, cut diagonally into thin slices
2 tbsp miso
2 stalks celery, with leafy tops, cut diagonally into thin slices
4 oz mushrooms, thinly sliced
4 scallions, trimmed and thinly sliced lengthwise
4–6 oz fresh bean sprouts
8 oz fresh spinach, washed and sliced
1 oz fresh parsley, finely chopped
two 10-oz blocks tofu, cut into cubes or strips

FOR THE SAUCE:
7 fl oz vegetable stock
2 fl oz soy sauce

2 tbsp rice vinegar
1 tbsp barley malt syrup

Break the ramen into a mixing bowl. Measure the water into a saucepan and place over medium heat. Place the carrots in a steamer over the water. Bring the water to the boil and steam the carrots for 3 minutes. Remove the pan from the heat: arrange the carrot slices in the bottom of a deep frying pan and dissolve the miso in the carrot water. Pour this water over the ramen in the bowl and leave for 10–15 minutes.

Carefully arrange the remaining vegetables, in the order in which they are given, in layers over the carrots. Drain the ramen and place over the vegetables; arrange the tofu on top. Place the frying pan over a high heat and, at the same time, combine the sauce ingredients in a small saucepan and heat to simmering. Immediately pour the sauce over the ingredients in the frying pan, bring to a boil, cover the pan, and reduce the heat from high to medium. Simmer for 5–7 minutes. Serve hot with steamed rice.

Marinated Tempeh

Serves 4
Preparation time 1 hour 30 minutes, plus 6–8 hours marinating

two 8-oz blocks tempeh, defrosted
5 cloves garlic, finely chopped
2 medium onions, chopped
1 tart apple, quartered, cored, and chopped
7 fl oz olive oil
7 fl oz cider vinegar
juice of 2 lemons
2 fl oz soy sauce
1 oz fresh ginger, sliced
2 tsp black peppercorns, crushed but not ground
1 tsp mustard seed, slightly crushed
12 whole cloves
one 3-inch piece of cinnamon

Cut the tempeh into 1-inch cubes and arrange in an oven dish. Mix the remaining ingredients together in a large jug. Stir well, then pour over the tempeh. Cover the dish and leave to marinate for 6–8 hours (ideal for making in the morning and cooking when you get home from work). You may, if you choose, let the tempeh marinate for up to 24 hours. Preheat the oven to 375°F and bake the tempeh for 1 hour. Serve hot over rice with steamed greens and sautéed carrots to accompany.

FOOD FACTOR 2: DON'T HESITATE TO VEGETATE

The second essential component of The Plant Program is to increase the amount of vegetables and fruit you consume, noting that vegetables are even more important than fruit. The official recommendation of five portions a day, especially when each portion can comprise a glass of (commercial) fruit juice, a tablespoon of dried fruit, or a small bowl of stewed fruit,[25] is in my view completely inadequate. The evidence is overwhelming that an abundant intake of fruit and vegetables can play an important role in reducing cancer incidence.[26] You must be careful, however—especially if you are on chemotherapy—to avoid having too much fruit containing strong acids such as citric or oxalic acid. Do not eat too many oranges, lemons, grapefruits, limes, or berries or too much rhubarb or you can develop cystitis or other symptoms of excess acid, including sore and painful joints. Eat apples and pears (which are especially good for the digestive tract and hence colon cancer), melons, peaches, apricots, and bananas, which are much less acid. Make sure they are fresh and ripe.

In the case of vegetables, do not eat too much spinach or too many beets or tomatoes at one time for the same reason. Otherwise eat as many vegetables, including salad vegetables, as possible. The list of anticancer chemicals identified in vegetables and fruit just keeps on growing. The investigation of plant chemicals pioneered by Lee Wattenberg of the University of Minnesota has identified many agents that protect against cancer in laboratory studies.[27] Perhaps this is hardly surprising. I have always wondered why I have never seen or heard of a plant with cancer despite all the chemicals we pour on them, so perhaps in the same way mankind discovered that some substances such as honey contain natural antibiotics because they do not readily "go rotten," we should have realized long ago that plants contain anticancer agents. Indeed, some of the latest chemo-therapeutic agents such as the taxanes, which are derived from yew trees, are effective against both advanced breast and ovarian cancers (but do not attempt to eat yew directly, as it is poisonous).

Most fruit and vegetables include such vitamins as beta-carotene (the precursor of vitamin A) and other carotenoids such as lycopene (especially rich in yellow and orange vegetables such as carrots, saffron, red and yellow peppers, and peaches) and vitamins C and E. All these vitamins act as antioxidants, removing free radicals, which can damage cell walls and cell DNA, from the body.

Free radicals are highly reactive molecules that typically have very short lifetimes. The best way to think of the effect of free radicals, which are powerful oxidizing agents, in our body is to imagine a pat of butter or a piece of meat or some nuts going rancid. This occurs because of a chemical process called oxidation. The chemicals in vegetables and fruit help to prevent oxidation—they keep our tissues from going rancid. The pigments in red, orange, and yellow fruit and vegetables—such as beta-carotene in carrots and peaches and lycopene in tomatoes (especially "baby" ones), pink grapefruit, or red grapeskins—are powerful anti-oxidants and may have other cancer-preventing properties. Garlic and brussels sprouts are especially rich in antioxidants.

Beta-carotene has long been suggested to be protective against several forms of cancer. Research reported from Israel in 1995 suggests that ly-copene (the main tomato carotenoid) is a more potent inhibitor of human cancer cell proliferation than beta-carotene.[28] In addition to its powerful antioxidant properties, it suppressed IGF-1-stimulated growth of mammary cancer cells. Research reported from Japan also showed that lycopene significantly suppressed breast tumor development in genetically suscep-tible mice, partly because it suppressed serum levels of prolactin and free fatty acids.[29] (Reading some of these papers strongly suggests to me that many scientists know the factors that promote breast cancer. Why have we not been told? See Chapter 7 for further discussion on this point.)

Plants, especially green leafy vegetables and newly sprouted shoots such as bean sprouts and alfalfa, also contain folic acid, which is involved in mak-ing the copies of the chromosomes carrying our gene sequences when cells divide. This is the very point at which mistakes that could cause cancer are likely to happen. A great deal of evidence suggests that most Americans' diets are deficient in folic acid.[30] Deterioration in the elderly has also been attributed to folate deficiency.[31] Cardiovascular disease is also being attributed to high circulating levels of homocysteine formed by the metabolism of a substance called methionine when levels of folic acid and vitamins B_6 and B_{12} are too low.[32] Indeed, throughout the West, women wishing to become pregnant are advised to take folic acid pills to avoid birth defects such as spina bifida in their babies. Surely we should *all* be eating a diet that has adequate quantities of folic acid without having to resort to taking pills. As discussed previously, some of the chemotherapeutic drugs used to disrupt breast cancer cells replace folic acid in cell division. I believe that it was drinking fresh juices high in folic acid as soon as I was able to after chemotherapy that helped me to recover so quickly and saved my hair from falling out. I drank about half a pint of green Granny Smith apple with fennel juice, about 50-50 apple-fennel, and about half a pint of carrot juice each and every day. I also ate lots of melon, which is especially rich in folic acid. People who were treated with me who took folic acid pills still lost their hair, but all the people I have persuaded to use juices have kept theirs. Beans, nuts, seeds, citrus fruits, and dark green leafy vegetables such as spinach also contain folic acid.

I have mentioned plant estrogens in the context of soy several times because of their protective effect on breast tissue. Plant estrogens are found in almost all fruit, vegetables, and cereals. Vegetables such as soy, lentils, peas, and beans are all legumes capable of fixing nitrogen from the air to make proteins and are rich sources of isoflavones. Typically Mediterranean, Latin American, and Eastern diets include large quantities of legumes, and it has been calculated that a typical Western diet provides only about 3 mg of isoflavones a day compared with the 30 to 100 mg a day in Eastern diets. Recently concern has been raised that phytoestrogens may be endocrine disrupters. Researchers at Saint Michael's Hospital in Toronto[33] therefore assessed the effects of soy foods. They concluded that soy consumption can reduce cardiovascular disease risk without increasing the risk of hormone-dependent (breast or prostate) cancer.

Red clover has particularly high levels of coumestans and, like chick peas (the basis of the Greek food hummus) and lentils, it contains all four important dietary isoflavones. Red clover, which can be bought from herbalists, is something I have started taking recently because I believe it to be protective against breast cancer. Sunflower seeds and alfalfa sprouts also contain substantial quantities of phytoestrogen compounds. Berries and whole grain and other cereal products are also important sources of phytoestrogens. According to Adlercreutz,[34] flaxseed, clover, sunflower, and sesame seeds are rich sources. All nuts contain relatively high amounts, especially peanuts. Among fruit, strawberries, cranberries, blueberries, and blackcurrants are rich sources (although apples, plums, and bananas contain practically no phytoestrogens). Vegetables such as pumpkin, zucchini, broccoli, carrots, and garlic are rich sources.

Phytoprogesterones in the diet may also be important in protecting against breast cancer. In his book *Natural Progesterone*, published by John Carpenter Publishing in 1996, Dr. J. R. Lee argues that breast and other problems, including premenstrual tension, fibroids, and weight gain, especially fat deposition at the hips and thighs, are caused by estrogen dominance over progesterone, which can become worse as women approach menopause. Dr. Lee suggests that the problem is mainly the result of poor nutrition. He recommends eating plenty of fresh vegetables, whole grains, and fruit, as unprocessed as possible and uncontaminated by insecticides, artificial coloring agents, preservatives, or other toxic ingredients. One of the richest sources of natural progesterone is wild yam or sweet potato, and soy and fennel contain both phytoestrogens and phytoprogesterones. Flaxseed, because of its high content of lignans, which are converted in the digestive tract into substances that help to regulate endocrine function, has been shown in experiments to have a significant and specific role in improving the progesterone-to-estrogen ratio during menstrual cycles of women.[35] Much research on flax has been carried out by the U.S. Food and Drug Administration, the National Cancer Institute, and the Canadian Food Protection Branch.[36] The recommendation is to take about one tablespoon a day of flaxseed in your diet for each 100 pounds of body weight (but be prepared to go to the bathroom more often!).

I also eat sprouted seeds, including soy, pumpkin and sesame (both rich in zinc), sunflower, alfalfa, and lentil. They are rich in vitamin C and other vitamins and minerals and high-quality proteins. Here's how to do it:

+ Use a container with some sort of drainage, such as a colander, strainer, mesh tray, or even a flowerpot with a cloth net over the hole. A jar with a piece of cheesecloth or muslin held in place around the top with a rubber band is perhaps the simplest and most effective. The size of the jar depends on how many seeds you are sprouting, but it should hold at least half a liter (about 2 pints).

+ Seeds can be bought from health food stores, where they are usually labeled "organic," and some supermarkets. Do *not* buy seeds from agricultural merchants—they may well be contaminated with seed dressing chemicals, which might be fatal if consumed. Use only the clean, whole ones and throw out the rest.

+ For every 100 ml (about one-fifth pint) the jar holds, use between two and three tablespoons of seeds. First they must be soaked in four times their own volume of water, ideally filtered or mineral water, until their bulk is doubled. This normally takes about eight hours, or overnight. After this time, pour off the water.

+ The sprout container should be kept in darkness—just throw a dish towel over the jar. The seeds must be rinsed two or three times a day through the muslin mesh of the jar. Make sure you drain them thoroughly each time by turning the container upside down, or the sprouts will rot.

+ Throw away any seeds that have not sprouted after two days. The rest will be ready to eat after four or five days. On the last day they can be put into the light, but only for a few hours or they will become bitter.

+ Most sprouts will need a final rinsing and draining before being put in the fridge in a covered container for storage. Some varieties, however, have loose husks that need to be removed. Place the sprouts in a large bowl of water and agitate until the husks float to the top. Then you can skim them off.

Vegetables and fruit also contain compounds, or their precursor chemicals, that have no known nutritional value but that have anticancer properties. They include indoles, isothiocyanates, dithiolthiones, and organosulfur components (some of which are thought to produce natural pesticides). About twenty years ago epidemiological studies showed that consumption of cruciferous vegetables (e.g., bok choy, broccoli, brussels sprouts, cauliflower), which contain dithiolthiones, was associated with a decreased risk of developing cancer. A synthetic dithiolthione called oltipraz has been shown to inhibit the development of tumors of the breast (and lung, colon, and bladder) in laboratory animals. Like other beneficial plant chemicals, it interferes with cancer development in several ways, including activating the liver enzymes that remove cancer-causing agents from the bloodstream.[37] Sulforaphane, an isothiocyanate that is also found in cruciferous vegetables and is responsible for their sharp taste, is also thought to prevent cancer by activating detoxifying enzymes in the liver. In rats it blocks the formation of chemically induced breast cancers. In addition, a compound called indo-3-carbinol, found in cruciferous vegetables, has been found to affect estrogen metabolism and hence to be especially protective against breast cancer. Recent research at Robert Gordon University in Aberdeen suggests that only raw broccoli offers any protective effect against colon cancer, as measured by the amount of DNA damage in colon cells from laboratory pigs.[38] It is suggested that cooking destroys glucosinolates, which are the precursors of isothiocyanates produced in the colon, which are the substances protective against cancer. The degree of cooking of the broccoli is not described, however. As indicated below, it is always best to eat vegetables that are as raw as possible (light steaming or stir-frying), although it is important to cook all meat and fish thoroughly.

Garlic and onions, chives and leeks (the allium family—*Allium sativum* is the Latin name for garlic) are important in helping to protect against cancer. They contain chemicals similar to those used in antiradiation pills (cysteinelike amino acids) and are particularly useful in reducing the effects of diagnostic X rays and radiation therapy in the body. They contain powerful antioxidants (active against free radicals, including those produced by anticancer treatments). Allicin, one of garlic's main biologically active components, is created when garlic is crushed; it has been shown to decrease breast cancer and prostate cancer cell proliferation in laboratory studies.[39]

In addition to allicin, garlic also concentrates other powerful antioxidants such as selenium and germanium, which neutralize the free radicals that are believed to promote tumor growth and atherosclerosis (clogging of the arteries). Research into cancer at universities in Pennsylvania and Texas has identified two other compounds active against cancer in crushed garlic: diallysulfide and S-allyl cysteine. The Weizmann Institute of Science in Israel has identified a molecular mechanism thought to be the basis for some of garlic's therapeutic effects. Current studies at the Memorial Sloan-Kettering Cancer Center in New York on the mechanism of action of chemopreventative chemicals derived from garlic indicate that it is effective against breast and prostate cancer, especially in the initial phases of cancer development, partly by improving the cell's ability to eliminate carcinogens and reducing the ability of carcinogenic chemicals to bind to DNA. Preliminary studies at the same center have indicated that garlic also prevents breast and prostate cancer cells from dividing thereby limiting the growth of tumors.[40] Garlic is also a natural antimicrobial agent active against a wide range of fungi, bacteria, and viruses, and it was used for these purposes in World War I. Many people worry about smelling of garlic, but if everyone eats it, no one notices!

One of the problems if you have active cancer is in consuming the amount of fresh fruit and vegetables needed to deliver adequate quantities of anticancer chemicals to the sites of the tumors. The best way to overcome this problem is to extract juices from the vegetables and fruits. This way, the active compounds are separated from the large mass of fiber that you would otherwise have to chew through, and the anticancer agents are made more biologically available to your body. Even if you do not like certain vegetables, you can hold your nose and simply drink the juice as if it were a medicine—and it is! Naturopaths and some doctors have been treating patients with fresh juices and raw food to improve their health since the nineteenth century. The therapy was pioneered in Germany and Switzerland before being used by health clinics worldwide. Famous pioneers include Father Kniepp, Dr. Kellogg, Dr. Max Bircher-Benner, and Dr. Max Gerson. To make the quantities of juices needed you must invest in a juicer (*not a liquidizer*). There are several available, but when I had cancer I found that the cheaper ones burned out fairly quickly, and I have had a juicer normally used in commercial juice bars for the past five years.

Carrot juice is good, but do not drink more than a half-pint glass a day or you may turn orange (I did—with orange palms and an orange mustache, which was described grandly by one of my doctors as carotenosis). Do not have too much cabbage juice either. Cabbage contains substances known as goitrogens that can cause problems with the thyroid gland if taken in too large quantities, especially if it is eaten raw. It increases the requirement for iodine, which is essential for good nutrition (see p. 165) and for which the main source in the diet is seafood. I made juice with green Granny Smith apples, celery, and fennel, with small amounts of watercress, the main green juice I drank every day when I was ill with cancer.

In addition to juices, you should have masses of fresh salads and vegetables. I cook vegetables by lightly steaming them (not by boiling and certainly not by boiling them to death, and on no account adding bicarbonate of soda) or just "sweating" them in a little extra-virgin olive oil (essentially cooking them for a few minutes without water). This is an especially good method of cooking spinach, which is delicious if a few onions are softened in the extra-virgin olive oil first.

I eat lots of vegetable soups. I just slowly soften vegetables in a little olive oil and then add boiling water and simmer. Finally I add a dollop of miso and some cubes of tofu (optional), adding some snippets of seaweed (optional), cress, or lettuce leaves just before serving.

One of the problems people complain of when they start to eat lots of fruit and vegetables is the number of times they have to go to the bathroom. Sorry, but that is what is supposed to happen—two to three times a day is normal, not two to three times a week! Also, by not suffering from constipation you will reduce your chance of suffering from hemorrhoids (piles) and other varicose veins. A good indication that your diet is correct is when your stools float rather than sink. You may also suffer from "wind," but don't worry; after a few weeks of the diet recommended here, the body will adjust and you will have no further problems with flatulence.

If you're thinking of cheating by drinking bottled or frozen juices instead of freshly made ones, there is simply no point. If you cut an apple it immediately starts going brown (because it has oxidized) and you need the green unoxidized juice. The same is true for all juices. If you buy commercial juices they will be far more oxidized and chemically far less potent as anticancer agents. They may also contain some type of preservative or have undergone some process to keep them going from rotten (just think about it; how else could carrot juice be sold weeks after it is prepared?), so they will be chemically changed. I have discovered people with colon cancer changing the diet I recommend by eating vegetable pills instead of raw vegetables and their juices! Experimental and observational studies have shown that this does not help. For example, in a study beginning in 1985, beta-carotene was included in two large long-term chemoprevention trials sponsored by the National Cancer Institute in the United States—the Alpha-Tocopherol (vitamin E) Beta-Carotene (ATBC) Lung Cancer Prevention Study and the Beta-Carotene and Retinal Efficiency Trial. Previous epidemiological studies had suggested that diets high in beta-carotene (for instance, from carrots) had reduced lung cancer incidence. In the trial studies, daily doses of beta-carotene in combination with either vitamin E (alpha-tocopherol) or vitamin A (retinol) were administered for several years to tens of thousands of people thought to be at high risk of developing lung cancer. What happened? The rate of lung cancer in those taking the pills increased in both trials![41]

Whole foods are a complex package of essential nutrients with many benefits that cannot be found in bottles of pills. Whole foods really are greater than the sum of their parts. For example, natural foods contain enzymes that help break down the components of the food. Hence bananas are rich in carbohydrates and contain amylase, a carbohydrate-splitting enzyme. Natural carrot juice contains all sorts of substances that work with beta-carotene. Foods generally contain hundreds or thousands of substances (many of which have yet to be studied) that may be important for health. It has been suggested that the difference between natural vegetables and commercial juices or pills is similar to that between paper and trees. Be like Chinese people and eat everything when it is as fresh and ripe as possible. Unfortunately, with the advent of supermarkets, food tends to be much older when we eat it. Also, we tend to make just one shopping trip a week rather than buying fresh food in season every day as we did when I was a child.

Organic Food and Pesticides

In the United States, organic regulations have been developed on a state-by-state basis—currently there is no national organic legislation. The U.S. Department of Agriculture attempted to develop national organic standards in 1998, but these standards would have permitted the use of genetically modified (GM) ingredients, sewage sludge, and irradiation in food labeled as "organic." These proposed standards were withdrawn for redrafting. In the United Kingdom, organically grown food has its origins in the work of Sir Albert Howard, who published *An Agricultural Testament* in 1940, advocating that Britain preserve the "cycle of life" and adopt "permanent agriculture" systems, using urban food waste and sewage to build soil fertility. The first person to apply the term *organic* to food production was the American J. I. Rodale in his 1942 publication *Organic Gardening and Farming*. In 1946 the young Lady Eve Balfour was inspired by Howard to set up the Soil Association, a pioneering organic farming charity that today is the major U.K. organic certification organization. In 1960 the Soil Association opened the first shop in the United Kingdom selling organic produce. Interest in organic farming grew throughout Europe and the United States during the environmentally aware 1960s. In 1974 the Soil Association established the United Kingdom's first set of Organic Food Standards, which formed the basis of the European Union regulation 2092/91, which lays down in detail how food must be produced, processed, and packaged to qualify for the description "organic." The regulation also specifies detailed criteria for the inspection and subsequent certification of food producers and processors.

Sometimes people who advocate organic food are dismissed as middle-class food fanatics with no rational or scientific basis for their concerns. I'd like to tell you why this caricature is wrong, and why it is so vitally important that you insist on as much high-quality organic food as possible.

Pesticides are chemical poisons used to control a pest or disease. They include *insecticides,* which kill insects, *herbicides,* which kill plants, *fungicides,* which kill fungal diseases, and many other *-cides* designed to kill everything from worms to birds. Pesticides, together with fertilizers and drugs for animals—known as a group as veterinary products—are called agrochemicals. The establishment view is that a relatively small percentage of cancers are attributable to pesticides, following an epidemiological analysis in 1981 by Doll and Peto, which indicated that not more than 2 percent of cancers were attributable to the use of man-made pesticides.[42] If this is accurate, it is still a lot of cancers. However, this estimate preceded our knowledge of the endocrine-disrupting behavior of certain chemicals, so it is likely to be an underestimate in the case of breast and prostate cancer. The major categories of synthetic pesticides include organochlorines, organophosphates, and triazine herbicides.

Many pesticides are made from organic chemicals. This is where some confusion can occur, because in connection with food, the word *organic* has a good meaning, but when it is used to describe a chemical pesticide, it has precisely the opposite sense. Indeed, it is the antithesis of life. Let me explain why.

There are just ninety-two naturally occurring chemical elements on Earth, ranging from light elements such as hydrogen and oxygen (which together form water) to very heavy elements such as lead, gold, and uranium. Everything you see around you (and much you can't see) is made up of various combinations of these ninety-two chemical elements.

Even more remarkably, every living thing, from the simplest of single-celled plants to the most complex species on the planet, is created from compounds of just *one* element—carbon.

Carbon is an extraordinary substance. It can combine with other elements to form a vast number of compounds. Some of the simplest molecules, which we use for food—sugar and starches—are called carbohydrates. (The name comes from the fact that carbon is combined with hydrogen and oxygen in the ratio of 2 to 1 as in water [hydrate]). Carbohydrates are used by life-forms mainly for energy and as an energy store. Fats, proteins, and vitamins are also organic or carbon-based chemicals. The chemistry of the unique chemical element carbon is the basis of all life—and because of their association with life, such chemicals are known as *organic* chemicals.

Organic chemical pesticides are potentially dangerous to us because they are based on the chemical wonder-element, carbon. Although they have been specially designed and configured to kill other animals or plants, the potential clearly exists for serious and profound disruption to occur within our own chemical life processes.

Since the end of the Second World War, industrialization of agriculture has been achieved by the increasing application of mechanization and the use of monocultures and of higher-yielding, more efficient crops and animals, with the application of an enormous range of pesticides to kill small organisms and a plethora of veterinary products to treat agricultural animals. The introduction of DDT during the Second World War marked the beginning of a very rapid growth in pesticide use, and other organochlorine pesticides—such as dieldrin and aldrin—were introduced in the late 1940s. Although environmental scientists have warned of the impact of such pesticides on wildlife for many years—for example, their effect on bird reproduction—the potential impact on humans, including endocrine disruption, is of increasing concern.

The use of DDT was banned in the United States in 1972, but it is still used in many developing countries. Other organochlorines such as aldrin and dieldrin, which are structurally similar to DDT, are no longer in general use in most developed countries. They share with DDT the common characteristics of a high degree of persistence in the environment, endocrine disruption, and the suspicion of carcinogenicity. What are we still using today that in the future we will find evidence to ban?

Organophosphates were first developed as nerve gas agents for chemical warfare in Britain, France, Germany, and the United States during the Second World War. They work by affecting nerve junctions. To fire a nerve impulse across a junction requires the body to produce a substance called acetylcholine. This must be broken down immediately after use by another chemical, an enzyme called acetylcholinesterase. Organophosphates prevent this substance from working properly by locking onto it. Hence the organophosphate pesticide is called an inhibitor. The locking-on is a two-stage process: the first is reversible, but the second—called aging—is not. So the nerve keeps firing. Organophosphates are implicated mainly in diseases of the nervous system rather than breast cancer, although recent work suggests that some of them are endocrine disrupters. Anyway, reducing exposure is desirable, especially in minimizing the depression accompanying breast cancer and its treatment.

According to Lang and Clutterbuck, animal studies have implicated about fifty pesticides as cancer-causing agents.[43] Many other pesticides are suspected of causing birth or genetic defects, and over sixty pesticides have been implicated in causing various reproductive effects. According to McMichael,[44] there has been a thirtyfold increase in global pesticide use and a ninefold increase in chemical fertilizer use since the 1950s. This has increased food yield, but it has also caused widespread chemical pollution, destruction of wildlife, and disturbance of ecosystems. As of the mid-1990s, U.S. agriculture used about 402,500 tons of pesticides per year, although even more than that, about 992,000 tons of insecticides, were used in nonagricultural applications, including forestry, landscaping, gardening, food distribution, and home pest control.

Insecticides and fungicides are the most important pesticides with respect to human exposure in food because they are often applied shortly before or even after harvesting. Herbicide use has also grown as chemicals have increasingly replaced traditional methods of cultivating land, such as crop rotation, in the control of weeds. Herbicides now account for two-thirds of agricultural pesticides.[45] Atrazine, a member of the s-triazine group of herbicides, is reported to be the most widely used herbicide in the world.[46] Exposure of breast cancer cells in tissue culture to atrazine leads to increased production of an estrogen metabolite, and it has been shown to cause mammary tumors when given in high doses to certain strains of laboratory rats.[47] The International Association for Research into Cancer (IARC, part of the World Health Organization) has concluded that there is limited evidence that atrazine is carcinogenic in animals, but it is a possible human carcinogen.[48] Atrazine is on the Environmental Endocrine Disrupters list of the U.S. Environmental Protection Agency and the World Wildlife Fund. Atrazine has been banned in several countries but is well established as a herbicide and widely used in the United States and Canada, leading to widespread regional water pollution. Another member of this group of herbicides is metrabuzin, which is also widely used on a variety of crops. They both work by inhibiting photosynthesis.

The alternative to this chemical nightmare is to buy organically produced food. Many farms or cooperatives now offer delivery of fresh organically grown produce. Even in the 1950s my father, who objected to the increasing use of chemicals to grow and process food, taught me to search for fruit and vegetables with grub holes in them on the basis that they would be less likely to contain pesticides. Prior to getting breast cancer, I had forgotten that advice.

If you can afford to do so, buy organically grown food, or at the very least buy organically grown potatoes and carrots. If you cannot afford organically grown produce and have a garden or access to one, grow your own. Salad vegetables in particular should be organically grown because they are eaten raw so the chemicals in them are not broken down at all by cooking. Otherwise, remove and discard the outer leaves of cabbage or lettuce, for example, and wash the rest in a weak solution of (cheap malt) vinegar, bought in glass, not plastic, bottles, before rinsing thoroughly and preparing in the normal way. This will not remove all chemicals now used in agriculture and horticulture (because many are systemic and hence occur throughout the plant), but it will reduce those sprayed directly onto the surface. Peel fruit if it is not organically grown (because unfortunately the skin, which is otherwise very nutritious, is often treated with chemicals and then waxed so the chemicals do not wash off). It is easy to see this from the way water runs off the surface of the fruit, just as if it were running off a plastic raincoat. This is often the case with oranges, grapefruit, and lemons and some heavily marketed commercial apples. Of course, it does not matter too much whether or not citrus fruit has been waxed if it is to be peeled, but it does if you are using it to make marmalade or other food that uses the skin or the rind of the fruit. I avoid eating apples that have been treated in this way. Just one important cautionary note: animal manure and waste is the main fertilizer universally used in organic farming, so pathogens will remain on your foods unless you are particularly vigilant and wash all fruit and vegetables thoroughly before eating them.

Cooking with Vegetables the Plant Way

Delicious Curly Kale

Serves 4
Preparation time 45 minutes

2 lb curly kale
1 tbsp olive oil
5 cloves garlic, chopped
1 large onion, thinly sliced
1 tsp freshly ground black pepper
½ tsp ground nutmeg
1 sweet red pepper, seeded and thinly sliced

Trim the kale and immerse it in cold, salty water for 5 minutes. Rinse each leaf under cold running water, slice into narrow pieces, and place in a colander. Heat the oil in a large saucepan over medium heat. Sauté the garlic and onion until clear and tender. Add the pepper and nutmeg and stir the sauté for 1 minute. Add the sliced kale and immediately cover the pan. Leave it cooking over medium heat for 5 minutes. Stir the kale so that the onion sauté is distributed through the greens, add the red pepper, and cover the pan. Cook over a low heat for 10 minutes. Stir well and serve immediately with rice, tempeh, and sautéed carrots or baked pumpkin.

Quick and Gorgeous Parsnip Soup

Serves 4
Preparation time 45 minutes

3 medium parsnips, peeled and chopped
1 large onion, chopped
3 stalks celery, chopped
2 tbsp olive oil
2 tbsp plain flour
2 pints soy milk
½ tsp freshly ground black pepper
¼ tsp salt
juice of ½ lemon
2 tbsp fresh parsley, chopped

Prepare the parsnips, onion, and celery. Heat the oil in a saucepan and add these vegetables to it. Stir well and sauté for 15 minutes over medium heat. When the vegetables are tender and golden, sprinkle the flour over them, stir, and gradually add the soy milk. Cook until the liquid is hot but not boiling, then pour the soup into a blender or food processor and liquidize to a smooth consistency. Return the soup to the saucepan and add the pepper and salt. Bring the soup to a simmer; add a little lemon juice at this stage to provide some sharpness. The consistency of the soup may be adjusted by adding vegetable stock or water. Let the soup simmer for 10 minutes and serve hot with parsley to garnish.

Cream of Spinach Soup

Serves 4
Preparation time 1 hour

1 lb fresh spinach, washed, trimmed, and chopped
1 tbsp olive oil
3 cloves garlic, finely chopped
2 medium onions, chopped

1 tsp freshly ground black pepper

2 tsp yeast extract

1 pint vegetable stock or water

2 tsp caraway seeds + 1 tbsp olive oil to sauté

1 tbsp plain flour *or* cornstarch

1 pint soy milk

1 tsp ground coriander

Prepare the spinach and leave in a colander to drain. Heat the oil in a large, deep saucepan over medium heat and sauté the garlic and onion until clear and tender. Add the pepper and stir for 1 minute. Stir in the yeast extract, then add the vegetable stock and bring to a low boil. Add the spinach, cover the pan, and reduce the heat. Let simmer gently for 3–5 minutes. Meanwhile, heat the other measure of oil in a saucepan and sauté the caraway seeds for 2 minutes. Sprinkle the flour over the oil and stir to make a thick paste (roux). Add the soy milk, a little at a time, stirring after each addition to make a sauce. Sprinkle the coriander over the sauce, stir well, and remove from the heat. Pour this sauce into the soup, stirring constantly as you do so. Add a little more stock if necessary to create the thickness of soup you enjoy. Serve hot with a garnish of coriander leaf.

Broccoli in Garlic and Almond Sauce

Serves 4

Preparation time 30 minutes

2 lb broccoli, trimmed and cut into florets

1 tbsp olive oil

1 whole head of garlic, peeled and chopped

1 tbsp fresh ginger, grated

½–1 tsp freshly ground black pepper

4 oz sliced almonds

1 bunch scallions, sliced into 2-inch lengths

Steam the broccoli for 5 minutes; leave the pan covered and put to one side, off the heat. Meanwhile, heat the oil in a large saucepan and sauté the garlic for 2 minutes, until just golden. Add the ginger and black pepper and stir for 1 minute. Add the almonds, scallions, and the steamed broccoli to the sauté, toss together, cover the pan, and leave over a low heat for 7–10 minutes. Serve hot as a side dish or over rice.

Arame and Vegetable Sauté

Arame is a Japanese seaweed, available in health food shops. This is a delicious dish that is easy to amend according to whatever vegetables you have at hand. You can make it a delicate little dish using one or two sautéed vegetables, or a huge and substantial one with half a dozen vegetables in the sauté. Try it very spicy with plenty of garlic and fresh chili or subtle and sloppy with a little extra broth thickened with arrowroot.

Serves 4
Preparation time 1 hour

2 oz dried arame
1 tbsp olive oil
4 oz mushrooms, sliced
5 scallions, sliced into 2-inch lengths
3 medium carrots, cut into small chunks
1 tbsp soy sauce
2 tbsp sesame seeds, roasted
freshly ground black pepper, to taste

First wash the arame to remove any grit, then soak it in plenty of water, in a bowl, for about twenty minutes. The arame will swell considerably. Lift the arame into a saucepan and pour fresh water over it. Place the pan over medium heat, make sure there is sufficient water to cover the seaweed, and bring to a boil. Immediately reduce the heat and simmer for 10 minutes, until the arame becomes very tender. Keep a close eye on it at this stage, as a great deal of froth is created initially and it can easily boil over. Meanwhile, heat the oil in a large pan and sauté the thinly sliced vegetables in it. Drain the tender arame and add to the vegetables. Stir the arame and vegetables over medium heat to mix the ingredients well. Season with soy sauce and cook for a few more minutes before serving hot. Serve over rice, sprinkling each serving with a teaspoonful of roasted sesame seeds and a little black pepper.

Classic Walnut and Red Cabbage Salad

Serves 4
Preparation time 30 minutes

4–6 oz walnut halves
1 small red cabbage, shredded
2 tart eating apples, quartered, cored, and chopped
1 small onion, thinly sliced
1 tbsp fresh parsley, chopped
3 cloves garlic, finely chopped
2 tbsp cider vinegar
3 tbsp olive oil
½ tsp dried marjoram
¼ tsp salt
½ tsp freshly ground black pepper

Mix the walnuts, cabbage, apple, onion, parsley, and garlic together in a large salad bowl. Blend the remaining ingredients together in a jar or jug and pour over the salad. Serve immediately, with a dollop of plain soy yogurt if desired. This salad will keep for 24 hours if chilled and stirred occasionally; its texture and flavor alter during this time. A variation involves finely chopping 2 slices of orange and tossing these in with the salad ingredients.

Roast Vegetables

+ Choose a large pan and coat well with olive oil.
+ Preheat oven to 350°F.
+ Wash a selection of your favorite vegetables and cut into large chunks or slices (e.g., eggplant, celery, zucchini, fennel, onions

[whichever sort you prefer], garlic, squash or pumpkin, different colored peppers, corn, tomatoes, asparagus). Place the vegetable pieces in a layer in the pan. Add your favorite herbs (e.g., parsley, thyme, rosemary, or basil) and then gently drizzle a few tablespoons of olive oil over the mixture, making sure the vegetables are coated evenly. Season to taste and put in the oven for one to one and a half hours. Baste a few times and serve with the juices.

+ Any leftovers can be used to make delicious sandwiches with the bread dipped or fried in the juices.

VEGGING OUT TO THE MAX:
Ten Key Ways to Boost Your Vital Vegetable Intake

If You Used to Do This . . .	Now Do This!
Boil your potatoes and cabbages to death	Buy an inexpensive stainless-steel "universal steamer." Place an inch of water in a saucepan, add the steamer, and fill it with veg. They take about the same length of time to cook, and you won't believe how much better they taste!
Think crudités meant only celery sticks dipped in salt	Keep the celery sticks but add raw carrot sticks, florets of raw broccoli and cauliflower, chunks of raw zucchini and sweet pepper, cucumber, tomato, scallions, and on and on. Ditch the salt, and if you have any room left on the plate, add a dollop of hummus or soy yogurt seasoned with chopped chives and herbs.

If You Used to Do This . . .	Now Do This!
Turn up your nose at any vegetable except frozen peas	Get real! And get an electric blender. Now lightly cook a huge mound of chopped veg in a little vegetable stock, push the whole lot through the blender, flavor with pepper and herbs, and serve. I call it Sneaky Soup because I always sneak great quantities of greens into it.
Think a salad was a careful arrangement of limp lettuce, shriveled cucumber, a slice of tomato, and half a boiled egg covered in creamy dressing	Aim to create a salad with at least five ingredients. Here is the "add list" for one of my favorite salads: grated carrot and turnip, chopped scallions, diced cucumber and zucchini, red kidney beans or tiny cubes of marinated tofu, watercress and parsley, radicchio and romaine lettuce. Mix and serve with sunflower seeds and a little walnut or sesame oil and a cider vinegar flavored with herbs drizzled over each serving.
Throw the parsley garnish away	Make sure it is fresh, then eat it with relish. If you have no relish, make some. Very finely chopped herbs, such as parsley, coriander, and watercress, and vegetables, such as tomato, onion, and zucchini, can be prepared quickly, mixed together, and served without a dressing. This will add valuable nutrients to your meal as well as a spot of color to your plate.

If You Used to Do This . . .	Now Do This!
Eat precisely one tablespoon of one vegetable at each evening meal	Well, that's a start. I used the Rainbow Rule to help me get into veg; here's how it works: fill one-quarter of your plate with white veg such as potato, parsnip, celery root, or turnip. These can be mashed, baked, roasted, or steamed. Fill the next quarter with orange veg such as carrot, sweet potato, or pumpkin; another quarter with yellow veg such as rutabaga, corn, or sweet pepper; and the final quarter with greens. You know what they are! Of course, you don't have to divide your plate into quarters— all these colors can be mixed and made into vegetable kebabs, roasted vegetable platters, salads, casseroles, stir-fries, and so on.
Think garlic was for rubbing inside salad bowls	Buy an enameled garlic crusher and a whole string of garlic. Whatever recipe you are reading, double the amount of garlic listed. Add chopped garlic to soups, stir-fries, and casseroles, and crushed garlic to salad dressings, hummus, and savory sauces.
Reach for a dictionary whenever you heard the word *brassica*	the cabbage family, then all the edible members of it that can become a part of your diet: broccoli, brussels sprouts, cabbages of all sorts, cauliflower, collards, kale, kohlrabi. These are the sulfur greens, rich in calcium and secondary components that are known to

If You Used to Do This . . .	Now Do This!
	be anticarcinogenic. Eat some raw or lightly steamed every day.
Think vegetable juice meant gravy and that a pound of carrots would last a year	Push one half pound of organic carrots, well scrubbed, through your new juicer. Drink immediately and go buy another pound of carrots. Tomorrow, add a couple of stalks of celery to the same juicing.

FOOD FACTOR 3: PROTEIN FOODS

I have put this as Factor 3 because of the difficulty many will find with living on a vegan diet, especially if they have not had breast or prostate cancer but wish to reduce their risk. I emphasize, however, that if you have active breast, prostate, or colon cancer you should eliminate *all animal products* until you are better.

After about eight months of eating only plant foods I began to feel "low." My doctors thought this was a reaction to what I had been through, but I realized that I was probably zinc-deficient. After iron, zinc is the next most important trace nutrient needed by our bodies.[49] It is involved in more than 200 enzymes in the human body, and deficiency in zinc is a common cause of depression. Zinc is essential for healing, so it is important that you have adequate zinc to help recover from surgery, radiation therapy, and chemotherapy. Its value has long been understood by ancient civilizations. When American doctors thought they had made a major breakthrough in identifying zinc levels as a crucial factor affecting recovery from burns and other injuries during the Vietnam War, it was pointed out that the remedy had been known to the ancient Egyptians and its use was recorded in the pyramids.

Many French doctors and every British vet I know is aware of how important zinc is, but I have yet to meet a British-trained doctor who is aware of its importance. In men its highest concentration in the body is in the prostate gland, suggesting that zinc is particularly important for its proper functioning. Zinc is also involved in cell division and in the way IGF-1 is controlled. Researchers at the University of Illinois have shown that a complex interactive set of factors are required to ensure that IGF-1 is active only when conditions are right for cell growth, and they describe a discrete role for trace nutrients—especially zinc—in regulating IGF-1 activity.[50] They have suggested that one of zinc's functions is to help inactivate IGF-1. New research also indicates that selenium may play a crucial role in prostate health. In one trial, men consuming higher concentrations of selenium (150 mcg/day) had three times less risk of prostate problems than men taking 86 mcg/day. One estimate suggests that the average intake of men in the United Kingdom is less than half that. Garlic is generally a good source of selenium.

Since I do not like taking zinc tablets (they can interfere with copper uptake and cause other problems—for example, taking too much can actually suppress the immune system) and because, at that time, I wasn't very knowledgeable about vegan food, I decided to introduce some meat into my diet because I knew that meat was a good source of zinc and selenium, but this was six months after all signs of cancer had disappeared (I would not have eaten meat if I had still had cancer). However, I buy only organically produced meat from specialist organic meat shops, which sell only meat raised using traditional and humane methods and without the use of chemicals such as antibiotics or other growth promoters. I eat only very small portions of "young" meat such as young lamb, pork, chicken, or duck, and game such as rabbit or venison. (Organically produced meat from beef cattle is also probably all right.) Game generally has higher levels of nutrients and far lower levels of fat than concentrate-fed animals, which have a sedentary life.

If I were an American, I would never eat beef or pork unless it was absolutely guaranteed to be organically produced. Growth hormone implants based on male and/or female hormones have been used extensively in beef production in America for about thirty years. According to the Institute of Agriculture and Natural Resources and the University of Nebraska, implants are available for all cattle except calves less than forty-five days old and breeding cattle. Some of the most potent hormone implants combine both male and female hormones. Such meat has higher levels of IGF-1 than untreated meat.[51] A genetically engineered pig growth hormone—porcine somatotrophin (PST)—is also available for purchase in the United States, but I can find no evidence of the use of such products in sheep meat production.

In an article in the Canadian press, Dr. Sonnenschein of Tufts University School of Medicine in Boston is quoted as saying, "it is very likely that hormone residue in American beef is a factor in the early onset of puberty among girls in recent decades. Early onset of puberty translates into higher risk of breast cancer."[52] It has been claimed that PST is safer than any of the steroid hormones banned by the European Union (but still used in America) because cooking destroys PST. However, this doesn't take IGF-1 levels into account, nor does it address the problem of uncooked or undercooked meat. Although the use of all such hormones is banned throughout Europe, on a BBC Radio 4 program, British pig farmers recently complained that European farmers were allowed to feed their animals on sewage sludge, which is forbidden in Britain! The message is clear. If you wish to eat pork, bacon, or ham (which are good sources of zinc), eat organically produced products.

The way the meat is cooked is important. My mother, who is a hearty 90-year-old, and all her generation of British women were taught to cook meat thoroughly, and that meant slowly. For all sorts of reasons, including preventing cancer, I will not now eat undercooked meat (however fashionable this is supposed to be) under any circumstances. Meat is a poor conductor of heat, and if it is not cooked properly, hormones in it (whether natural to the animal or introduced by man) will not be destroyed. Even if it is well cooked, steroid hormones such as those used in the United States, which include estrogens, may survive. Cooking meat so that it is burned on the outside and raw on the inside is bad for health generally. Cancer-promoting chemicals (heterocyclic amines [HCA], the most abundant of which is known as PhiP) are likely to be formed in the burned parts (burned meat has been implicated in colon cancer), while cancer-promoting chemicals including hormones will remain intact in the relatively raw meat inside. I never eat meat that could contain ground-up dairy animal, such as hamburger or sausages. Remember, official figures show that dairy cow meat contains even more IGF-1 than milk. Amounts of HCA range from very low levels in poached, steamed, or stewed meat and fish to very high levels in flame-broiled meat. PhiP has been linked to colon, prostate, and breast cancer.[53] High levels of HCA also occur in pan-fried meat.[54]

Other good sources of protein and essential trace nutrients such as zinc include eggs—zinc is concentrated in the yolks (but eat only organically produced eggs). Eggs also contain high levels of the amino acid cysteine used in antiradiation pills, so in moderation, egg consumption will help combat the effects of radiation therapy and diagnostic X rays. The sulfur in cysteine is in a form thought to deactivate free radicals and thus protect cells.[55] I ate one small organically produced egg a day while being treated with radiation therapy; I often eat organic eggs now, but never more than one a day. Otherwise, good sources of zinc include crabs, snails, and oysters (especially Atlantic oysters) or, if you are a vegan, sesame seeds (best as tahini—a delicious spread made from sesame seeds), pumpkin seeds, sunflower seeds, or wheat germ. Brewer's yeast is a particularly good source of many trace elements, including selenium, chromium, and zinc, and B vitamins, which are essential for the skin and nerve tissue (remember that breast tissue is a specially modified type of tissue related to skin tissue).

Fish and shellfish (ideally fresh, unfarmed, and unsmoked) are an excellent source of protein, but only cold water fish such as mackerel and salmon also contain concentrations of "good fats" known as omega-3 oils (see p. 173). Indeed, a Canadian scientist has recently suggested that the human brain could not have evolved unless we had access to the large omega-3 resources of shellfish and other coastal food sources. The coastal zone is typically where nutrients become concentrated at the interface between freshwater from land and saltwater. It is unfortunate that in Britain and many other industrialized countries the same processes that are designed to concentrate nutrients in estuaries and the coastal zone are concentrating pollutants, so that I no longer feel able to eat nutritious foods such as certain shellfish unless I can be sure they are from an unpolluted source.

Populations such as the Eskimos living on a predominantly fish diet have long been known to have less breast cancer than those eating other animal fats. If properly cooked, seafood also contains lots of iodine, and iodine compounds (like those of zinc) are involved in ensuring that mistakes (which could cause cancer) do not occur during cell division in the body.[56] After the thyroid, the highest concentration of iodine in human females is in the breast, suggesting that—as in the case of zinc, which is concentrated in the prostate in males—it plays an essential role in the proper functioning of breast tissue. (Indeed, I have helped many of my friends who had sore breasts before a period to overcome the problem by taking Icelandic kelp tablets.) Also, iodine has been shown to lower the incidence of breast cancer in menopausal laboratory rats.[57]

As a chemical element, iodine has very unusual behavior. It is called a conservative element, which means that it prefers to stay in water, and hence in Earth's system it ends up being concentrated in the oceans. This is why one of the main dietary sources is seafood. The distinctive chemistry of iodine means that it is easily lost when growing, processing, and cooking food (Chinese people tend to cook fish in sealed containers and use the juices to make soup, which keeps levels of iodine intake higher). Pasteurization of milk destroys up to 20 percent of available iodine, and several components of our diet contain compounds called goitrogens that increase our need for iodine. The plant called rape, from which rapeseed or canola oil is obtained, contains goitrogens, and to be on the safe side I avoid this in my diet and anything that contains unspecified vegetable oils, since they could include such oil.

To ensure that I have enough iodine I take kelp tablets. All seaweed has high concentrations of iodine and other nutrients, but it can also concentrate pollutants, including some radioactive isotopes that are in waters offshore of nuclear plants. I therefore eat only Icelandic kelp (because Iceland has a low population, uses only natural geothermal energy, and is farther away from most pollutant sources than any other supplier of seaweed that I can think of) Earlier in this century fish waste and seaweed were commonly used as fertilizer, but these have now been mostly replaced by inorganic fertilizers, including rock phosphate, which generally have low iodine content (but which can be rich in the radioactive element uranium and in the potentially toxic element cadmium, depending on the source).

Soils in most Western countries tend to contain much-reduced levels of organic humus because of industrialized farming, so they cannot effectively trap the iodine delivered to them in rainwater. Hence, crops now generally contain relatively low levels of this essential nutrient, making a natural supplement such as kelp important. Taking kelp in my diet has improved my skin enormously. If I run out of tablets for any length of time, my skin becomes rough, initially around my elbows, knees, and buttocks, and the roughness gradually extends over progressively larger areas until I take kelp again, when the roughness retreats. Seaweed also protects against radiation. Alginate, a mucous material extracted from seaweed, is used as a standard protective agent against radioactivity. Hence kelp and other seaweeds help reduce the side effects of X rays and radiation therapy. Agar-agar, which is widely used to replace gelatine in vegan foods, can also be used in your diet as a source of iodine. Other seaweeds that I use occasionally include arame, hiziki, dulse, and wakame. After softening in cold water for about 20 minutes, add to soups or stews immediately before serving (to preserve the iodine). Nori, which is commonly sold in sheets, can be used to wrap rice balls, sushi, and many other foods.

An extra bonus is that iodine is good for the brain. Iodine deficiency is the world's most common cause of mental retardation and brain damage.[58] Indeed, the untreatable condition known as cretinism, whereby children are born severely mentally retarded, can be caused by the mother's deficiency in iodine during pregnancy.

Cereals are a good source of protein and are discussed further under Food Factor 6 (see p. 183).

Another good protein source is nuts. I eat lots of nuts (but never preshelled because they quickly become rancid). I avoid uncooked peanuts and other groundnuts because they are sometimes naturally contaminated with microorganisms that produce cancer-causing chemicals known as aflatoxins. I boil or toast all ground nuts before eating and they taste delicious. I avoid brazil nuts, which can contain elevated levels of the radioactive substance radium 226. When one of my colleagues told me this because he was concerned that I was eating so many brazil nuts, I did not believe him. After leaving some of the nuts I had been eating in our detector overnight, I did!

PREVENTION FOR ORDINARY MORTALS

For those without breast cancer who wish to cut their risk or those who have recovered from breast cancer (like me). Remember to keep total animal products to no more than 15 percent of calories each day.

If You Used to Do This . . .	Now Do This!
BREAKFAST	
Eat processed refined cereals with milk and white sugar	Have organic muesli with a tablespoon of flaxseed, moistened with fruit juice previously sweetened with honey, raw cane sugar, or molasses, or use rice, soy, or coconut milk.
Eat fried sausage, bacon, scrambled eggs, and fried bread	Have one of the following: 1. Grilled organic bacon or vegetarian alternative, tomatoes and mushrooms brushed with, or softened in, olive oil. Toast or lightly fry bread in olive oil. 2. Haddock poached in 50 percent soy milk and 50 percent water topped with a poached organic egg. 3. Boiled or poached eggs on whole-grain organic bread lightly fried in olive oil.
Have toasted white bread and butter with marmalade	Have toasted organic whole-grain bread with Granose soy spread and marmalade
Drink commercial orange juice	Drink freshly made melon and raspberry juice or apple juice or any alternative juice you enjoy.
SNACKS AND NIBBLES	
Nosh on commercial cookies, especially those containing dairy	Choose dried fruit, nuts, pumpkin seeds, bananas, dried coconut, dairy-

If You Used to Do This . . .	Now Do This!
(e.g., whey, casein, lactose, milk powder)	free sesame bars, or other snacks from health food stores.
Use cheesy or yogurt-based dips	Use hummus, tahini, or taramasalata.
Enjoy a late-night milk chocolate or malt drink	Check the label, then make it with soy milk instead of dairy, using raw sugar, vanilla, or other flavorings you enjoy.

MAIN MEALS

Cook meat in butter or lard and eat it rare or undercooked	Roast or grill meat slowly and thoroughly using olive oil, sea salt, black pepper, and other herbs for flavor. Eat only small portions. Roast potatoes in the juices, and then use juices to make the gravy.
Eat hamburgers, sausage, pâté, and prepared dishes from supermarkets	Eat veggie burgers or vegetarian sausages. Fish or eggs are the ultimate fast food. Steam or poach fish in water or white wine flavored with ginger, onions, fennel, or dill or simply grill after brushing with olive oil and seasoning with salt, black pepper, and herbs.
Eat canned peas	Lightly steam fresh peas, snow peas, asparagus, broccoli, or any other vegetable and keep the juice to make soup or gravy. Don't add butter; use olive oil flavored with herbs.
Eat French fries, buttered or roast potatoes, baked potatoes with butter or cheese	Scrub potatoes before baking or steaming, then rub in olive oil and garnish with chopped parsley before serving. Eat baked potatoes with hummus or taramasalata instead of butter and cheese.
Enjoy milky sauces and cream soups	In sauces, replace the milk with soy milk; in soups, substitute as in the cream of spinach recipe on p. 155.

If You Used to Do This . . .	Now Do This!
Serve thin soups	Serve miso-based soups (p. 131) or simple vegetable broth.
Eat rich desserts	Choose from fresh fruit salads, baked bananas, water ices or sorbets, soy ice cream or the tofu fruit desserts described in Food Factor 1, caramelized oranges, pears stewed in red wine, baked apples filled with dried fruit and chopped nuts. Use soy cream and adjust the taste with fruit juice, honey, or raw sugar and a few drops of organic vanilla essence.
	A wonderful orange sauce made with the juice of two oranges gently heated with raw sugar (to taste) and a few drops of vanilla (with a teaspoon of Cointreau) can be poured over many desserts before serving, making them even more delicious.
Serve a cheese course	Substitute a salad course with pine nuts, sun-dried tomatoes, herb-flavored olives, artichoke hearts, and marinated tofu.
Use commercial mayonnaise or salad dressing	Make a base of 3-to-1 virgin olive oil to wine, cider, raspberry, or balsamic vinegar, season with a pinch of raw sugar, sea salt, and black pepper to taste, and use English or French (Dijon) mustard, various herbs, and garlic to ring the changes.
Serve after-dinner chocolates	Buy the organic, dairy-free, dark chocolate version.
Drink milky tea or coffee	Substitute from lists in Food Factors 1 and 7.

FOOD FACTOR 4: OILS AND FATS

Many people are confused about the type and quantity of oils and fats they should be eating. Also, we have been persuaded to buy lots of spreads based on (usually altered and processed) polyunsaturated fats. Our bodies do need fats, but only in the quantities and forms that we would have consumed as hunters or gatherers.

Fats are solid at room temperature, oils are liquid. However, scientists often use the term *fat* to include all oils and fats, whether they're solid or liquid. Chemically, fats are made up of three molecules of fatty acids and one of an alcohol called glycerol. The word *triglycerides* is also used to describe fat—it means three (*tri*) fatty acid molecules plus glycerol—triglyceride.

Fatty acids are simply acids that are found in fats. There are four major fatty acids: palmitic, stearic, oleic, and linoleic. Remember, each molecule of fat contains three of these four fatty acids. It's the *combination* of these acids in the fat molecule that determines whether the fat is saturated, unsaturated, or polyunsaturated—words we've all heard a great deal in the past few years. Let me explain them.

Lipids (fats and oils), which are made from various combinations of fatty acids combined with glycerol, have long tails of carbon atoms (often fifteen to seventeen carbon atoms) combined with hydrogen. Some fatty acids are chains of carbon atoms attached by single bonds, and all their spare bonds are attached to hydrogen. They are called saturated (with respect to hydrogen). Some have double bonds between carbon atoms and are called unsaturated. Unsaturated fatty acids can have one (monounsaturated) or many (polyunsaturated) double bonds between carbon atoms. Double bonds make fatty acids and lipids melt more easily; hence most oils are unsaturated, while fats, especially animal fats, which are generally saturated, are solid at room temperature. In nature, fats serve an important role in storing energy (they store more energy than the same mass of carbohydrates) and as an insulator against heat loss. The way the carbon and hydrogen are assembled means that these substances are generally insoluble in water and are said to be hydrophobic.

Saturated

Palmitic fatty acid has sixteen carbon atoms and no unsaturated carbon bonds, so it's called "saturated." Stearic fatty acid has eighteen carbon atoms and no unsaturated carbon bonds, so it's also called "saturated." Saturated fat is known to raise the level of cholesterol in your blood. The more you eat, the higher your cholesterol level and the greater your chances of suffering a stroke or heart attack. Animal fat—lard, butter, and the fat contained in meat—contains lots of saturated fat. A few plant fats also contain significant amounts, principally coconut and palm oil. Among all the controversies about fats and oils, the message to minimize saturated fat in our diet has remained unchanged for more than thirty years.

Monounsaturated

Oleic fatty acid has eighteen carbon atoms and one unsaturated carbon bond, so it's called "monounsaturated." Ongoing research suggests that monounsaturated fat is much healthier than saturated fat. Experiments on humans show that switching to monounsaturated fat from the saturated kind can not only decrease the risk of heart disease but may also be able to lower your blood pressure. A major source is olive oil. This contains more than 80 percent monounsaturated fats and is naturally resistant to oxidation, which means it is relatively safe for cooking and is also less prone to rancidity than other types of unsaturated fat. Rancidity is believed to promote cancer.

Polyunsaturated

Linoleic fatty acid has eighteen carbon atoms and two unsaturated carbon bonds, so it's called "polyunsaturated." Early research indicated that polyunsaturated fats lowered total and LDL cholesterol (low-density lipoprotein—the "bad" form of cholesterol) more than monounsaturated fats. The latest research, however, finds no difference in their cholesterol-lowering ability. However, the more polyunsaturated an oil is, the more it can be damaged by heat, air, and light. Most polyunsaturated oils should only be used raw because once damaged they form free radicals. Good sources of polyunsaturated fats include sunflower and corn oil. We all need a little linoleic acid in our diets every day because, of the four major fatty acids, this is the only group our bodies cannot synthesize.

Essential Fatty Acids

The two classes of essential fatty acids (EFAs), which are polyunsaturated and which you will undoubtedly have heard about, are named omega-6 and omega-3. They are both necessary for good health because they provide the catalysts for various metabolic functions (e.g., the synthesis of prostaglandins, which are important as cell regulators and for the proper functioning of the immune system). Through a complicated transformation process, EFAs become biologically active and therefore become useful links in many metabolic systems. They are called "essential" because the body cannot make them and they must be obtained from food sources. Most vegetable oils provide the EFAs to a greater or lesser extent, but they are not significantly present in meat.

+ Omega-6 fatty acids (e.g., linoleic acid) are found in vegetable seeds and the oils produced from them. Good sources include oils made from safflower, sunflower, corn, soy, evening primrose, pumpkin, walnut, and wheat germ.
+ Omega-3 fatty acids (e.g., alpha linolenic acid) are found in cold water fish such as salmon, mackerel, and sardines and are also found in linseed (flaxseed), evening primrose, borage seed, and soybean oil. In addition to being protective against breast cancer, they are considered protective against a range of other conditions, including coronary heart disease and high blood pressure, arthritis, eczema and psoriasis, and benign prostatic hyperplasia (enlarged prostate).[59] The food supplement spirulina (a microscopic algae) contains both linoleic and linolenic acids.

Japanese researchers have shown that a deficiency of these essential fatty acids leads to an impaired ability to learn and recall information. Gamma linoleic acid (GLA) is a particularly good omega-3 fatty acid, which is enriched in organ meats such as liver (but eat only from organically reared animals) and in evening primrose oil (but do not have this in gelatine capsules, which are made from rendered dead animal carcasses).

It has been suggested that the amount of omega-6 oil in most Western diets is about twenty times that of omega-3 oil.[60] The advice now is to take no more than 10 percent of daily calories in polyunsaturated fats, with about a seven-to-one ratio of omega-6 to omega-3. I do eat lots of fish, but I am prepared to pay for wild rather than farmed fish since they are less likely to contain antibiotic residues and other man-made pollutants. However, I do not take fish oils, because of concern that they can contain concentrations of pollutants such as organochlorine pesticides and PCBs (see p. 219). Fish are also rich in vitamin D, essential for healthy bones and suggested by research at Harvard University in the United States and Saint George's Medical School in London to help prevent breast cancer.[61] Vitamins A and D may work to reduce risk by lowering blood levels of IGF-1.[62]

I will no longer eat dairy products in any guise, and I rely mainly on first-pressed extra-virgin olive oil for everything from cooking to salad dressings. This is more than 80 percent monounsaturated fatty acids and naturally resistant to oxidation, which means it is relatively safe for cooking. However I never reuse the oil, and I cook food slowly so that the oil is not damaged and the food absorbs the flavor.

The only oils I use have been organically grown and extracted by cold pressing. There are three methods of extraction:

+ Cold pressing. This is the traditional hydraulic pressing process in which the temperature is kept low throughout and therefore preserves temperature-sensitive vitamins. The end product is expensive, mainly because there is a high percentage of waste in the discarded pulp, but the oil is nutritious and tastes and smells good. It may be more expensive, but you consume less.

+ Screw or expeller. This process involves high-pressure pressing, which generates high temperatures. Vitamins are destroyed during this process, and although it enables more oil to be extracted, it is dark and strong-smelling and needs further refining and deodorizing.

+ Solvent extraction. This is the most common process used because it produces the highest yields. The grains or seeds are ground, steamed, and then mixed with solvents. The solvents used are either the petroleum-based benzene, hexane, or heptane. The mixture is then heated to remove the solvents and then washed with caustic soda. This has the effect of destroying the oil's valuable lecithin content. After this it is bleached and filtered, which removes precious minerals as well as any colored substances. Finally it is heated to a high temperature to deodorize it. One other aspect of vegetable oils produced by solvent extraction is that they have lost their vitamin E. This vitamin helps prevent the oil from going rancid. Rancid oils are damaging because they provide the raw material for producing free radicals in our bodies. Sometimes chemical retardants are added to stop the oil from turning rancid, but it would seem to be much more sensible to stick with the cold-pressed oils, which can keep well, if properly stored, for up to six months.

All oils should be stored in dark opaque stoppered glass bottles to minimize oxidation and used cold in salad dressings or by the teaspoonful. I never use oils from plastic bottles, since many of the potentially harmful chemical substances in plastics are fat-soluble. In keeping with my general philosophy of eating whole unprocessed foods as much as possible, I obtain my oils as part of the total food: for example, I eat fish for fish oils, and flaxseed for flaxseed oil. The benefits of this approach can be demonstrated in relation to flax: according to Ingram and others,[63] it is flaxseed—but not flax oil—that is rich in the lignan precursors that are anticarcinogenic. Flaxseed or linseed may be particularly helpful against breast cancer and is also excellent for avoiding constipation and hence piles and varicose veins.[64] Research by Dr. Lillian Thompson of the University of Toronto reported in 1999 showed that a lignan precursor from flaxseed reduces the growth rates of existing breast cancer by more than 50 percent. It has also been shown to be protective against colon cancer. Flaxseed is an abundant source of lignan precursors, which are thought to be changed by the action of bacteria in the human intestine to compounds extremely protective against breast cancer. Lignans are also antioxidants, antibiotic, and antitumorigenic. The only oil in my diet that I do not obtain from whole food is cold-pressed extra-virgin olive oil. I eat no butter and no margarine.

In many Mediterranean restaurants it is usual to have virgin olive oil flavored with herbs to dip bread into. It is so much tastier and healthier than butter. I do this now if I have dinner parties. Usually my guests eat their bread dipped in flavored olive oil with great relish. I cannot remember anyone complaining or asking for butter. On the contrary, I have noticed that many of them have adopted the idea. The Spanish, Italian, and Greek people I know use olive oil with fish or tomato paste and salad, for example, to make sandwiches, instead of butter or polyunsaturated spreads on their bread. This is not only healthier, but the sandwiches and snacks are much more delicious than those most people in the United States or the United Kingdom eat.

Even though the health risk is low, I avoid rapeseed or canola oil. Canola has been bred from old varieties of rapeseed in Canada and is reported to contain very low levels of erucic acid. Although canola is a heart-healthy oil, when a diet high in the oil derived directly from the original rapeseed is fed to laboratory animals, it is suspected of having a pathogenic effect.[65] Canola oil is now the most widely consumed food oil in Canada and is approved by the U.S. Food and Drug Administration, but I believe olive oil is a better choice.

I also avoid products containing vegetable oils where the type of oil is unspecified since they could contain rape, canola, palm, or coconut oil. I avoid all margarines including those claiming to be high in polyunsaturates, because they have been hydrogenated (which involves passing hydrogen gas through them under pressure, often in the presence of a nickel catalyst). This process can produce "trans fats," which some nutrition experts believe are unhealthy and which have been implicated in breast cancer.[66] The Western diet typically contains large quantities of trans fatty acids (TFAs), originating primarily from hydrogenated fats, which experimental evidence suggests impair essential fatty acid metabolism.[67] TFAs are somewhat similar in structure and behavior to saturated fatty acids, and the World Health Organization recommends that manufacturers reduce the levels of TFAs arising from hydrogenation.

OIL YOU NEED TO KNOW:
Ten Ways to Modify Your Fat Intake

If You Used to Do This . . .	Now Do This!
Spread your toast with a thin layer of butter, wait until it soaked in, then cover it with a thick layer of peanut butter	Leave out the butter.
Spread your toast with a thick layer of butter or margarine	Drizzle a little organic cold-pressed extra-virgin olive oil over your toast instead. It tastes delicious . . . really!
Buy oil labeled canola or unspecified vegetable oil	Buy only cold-pressed extra-virgin organic olive, walnut, sesame, or sunflower oils.
Prepare a fondue every weekend	Keep the little forks, but switch ethnic loyalties and prepare a platter of raw and steamed vegetables surrounded by a selection of Thai, Japanese, and Chinese dips and sauces.
Buy a cheese and pickle sandwich from your local deli every lunchtime	Buy a tub of their hummus instead, along with a salad and some pita bread to dip into it.
Buy crackers and snack foods without reading the labels	Read all labels for fat content! And don't leave your spectacles at home. I suggest you buy matzos to put in your cracker barrel and buy fresh and dried fruit instead of snacks.
Insist on making popcorn before you watched that film	Go ahead, but use an air-popper to make it. They make a good gift and require no fat. Add salt or your favorite spices as usual.

If You Used to Do This . . .	Now Do This!
Order the Four Cheeses pizza	Try the pizza without the mozzarella but with extra olives, capers, mushrooms, garlic, etc.
Order baked potato with butter, chili con carne, and cheese sauce	Order baked potato with baked beans or hummus and a side salad.
Go crazy for any dessert topped with cream	Dig out a recipe for orange sauce (p. 170), or keep a small bottle of organic maple syrup in your cupboard, and drizzle a little over your favorite nondairy dessert.

FOOD FACTOR 5: SEASONING AND FLAVORINGS

Healthy food doesn't have to be—indeed, *shouldn't* be—bland food. Until recently the main methods of preserving food were to add lots of salt, especially to meat and vegetables, sugar to fruit, and alcohol to a range of products. It has been said that the British, because they shipped so much food from their overseas territories, developed a particular liking for these tastes. Food naturally contains sodium, so we do not need to add any to our food. Overuse of salt and sodium bicarbonate have been linked by Gerson to cancer, and it continues to be implicated by some researchers in promoting certain types of cancer, including nasopharyngeal (nose and throat) cancer.

It is easy to learn to change your taste, and you will find that food tastes much better, with far more subtle flavors, when salt is not added. Eastern people consume lots of salt in soy sauce, so I do not think it is one of the most critical things to do in combating breast cancer, but it is helpful to your health generally, and I recommend that you reduce your salt and refined sugar intake as much as you can, as soon as you can.

I grow fresh herbs such as parsley, thyme, chives, marjoram, rosemary, and mint in a small patch in the garden and buy others from the supermarket. Herbs are good for you and help to make food taste delicious. I did not use spices when I was ill, but the Chinese do use spices, especially in Szechwan and Hunan provinces. Also, Korean and Thai food is very heavily spiced yet breast and prostate cancer rates there are low. Hence despite the recommendations in many anticancer-diet books, I do not believe that spices are a primary factor in the incidence of breast or prostate cancer.

On the other hand, I never eat the horribly colored pink or yellow food now sold as Eastern food in some shops, restaurants, and supermarkets, although real saffron made from crocus stamens and traditionally used to color rice yellow contains carotenoids and has anti-free-radical properties.

I use vinegar (wine or cider, preferably organically produced) with organic extra-virgin olive oil as the basis for delicious salad dressings. I never eat commercially produced mayonnaise or other such glop.

Unrefined sugars or molasses are fine (although check that you really are buying raw sugar, as some brown sugar is white sugar dyed with caramel, or burned sugar). I also eat honey (preferably wild honey from unpolluted sources). Refined white sugar (called pure white and deadly by some) is just empty calories stripped of nutrients. I never eat it, but molasses or raw brown sugar is fine. Traditionally, the Chinese and Japanese have eaten very few sweets. Their treats, including those for small children, were pumpkin seeds or dried fruit.

Some Spicy Ways to Enliven Any Dish

Garam Masala
....

This mixture may be changed to suit your taste. Use a mortar and pestle, a hand-turned pepper mill, or an electric grinder, such as a coffee grinder, to grind your spices. It is best, and noticeably different in flavor and aroma, to use whole spices, grinding them only when you need them. We all have need for little shortcuts now and again, however, so simply store any surplus ground spices in a labeled airtight jar in a dark cupboard.

Makes 2–3 tbsp, enough for 1 dish
Preparation time 5 minutes

2 tsp freshly ground coriander
1 tsp freshly ground black pepper
1 tsp freshly ground cumin
½ tsp freshly crushed cardamom
½ tsp freshly ground cloves
½ tsp freshly ground cinnamon

If you can, grind these spices individually, measure them, then mix them.

Mild and Fresh Spice Blend

This mixture can be used to flavor soups, stews, and other dishes; adjust it to suit your taste.

Makes 3–4 tbsp, enough for one dish
Preparation time 10 minutes

1 tbsp caraway seeds
3 cloves garlic, crushed
2 tsp fresh ginger, grated
1 tsp freshly ground black pepper
1 tsp ground coriander
½ tsp salt
¼ tsp ground allspice

Grind all the ingredients in a mortar and pestle until the caraway seeds are slightly crushed. Stir into the dish, either during the sauté or shortly before serving, and adjust to taste.

Warming Spice and Herb Blend

This is a more robust blend, which may be used alone or in combination with the above recipe in savory dishes. The ingredients may be adjusted to suit your taste.

Makes 5 oz, enough to serve 4
Preparation time 15 minutes

5 scallions, finely chopped

3 cloves garlic, finely chopped

1 tbsp fresh ginger, grated

1–2 fresh hot chilies, finely chopped

2 tbsp fresh basil, chopped

1 tsp freshly ground cardamom

1 tsp freshly ground black pepper

¼ tsp ground nutmeg

Blend all the ingredients and add to the dish during the sauté.

LIVELY SPICES:
Ten Healthy Ways to Excite Your Tastebuds

If You Used to Do This . . .	Now Do This!
Sprinkle everything with salt	Stop cooking with salt. Try seasoning your meal with tamari (wheat-free soy sauce) or gomasio, a mixture of ground sesame and sea salt.
Spread yeast extract on your toast	Good idea, but on alternate days spread miso on your toast for the similar-but-different flavor and the added nutrient value it brings.
Serve boiled carrots with a dollop of butter	Steam the carrots, then toss them in a light sauté of garlic and/or freshly grated ginger.
Think black pepper was the only spice	Arrange a small collection of spicy condiments on the table including black pepper, chili pepper flakes, and Tabasco sauce. Visit your local ethnic grocer to explore a new world of spices. Then begin to experiment . . .
Use mayonnaise and nothing else on every salad you were given	Mix finest olive oil with an herb-flavored cider vinegar, freshly crushed

If You Used to Do This . . .	Now Do This!
	garlic, and a little mustard. Or drizzle a little freshly squeezed lemon juice and sesame or walnut oil over your salad. A splash of Tabasco will lift the flavor to the roof.
Think potatoes were only there to soak up the gravy	Steam potatoes and cabbage, then toss them gently in a light sauté of caraway seed and chopped garlic. Season with good old black pepper to taste.
Think every soup needed a hefty dose of beef broth and monosodium glutamate (MSG) to be tasty	Make your soups with a strong vegetable broth including the seaweed kombu, which has flavoring and thickening properties similar to MSG.
Think all vinegar was white and only good for making your lips pucker	Buy the finest organic cider vinegar and organically grown fresh herbs and put the two together in the prettiest bottle you can find. Try tarragon, rosemary, basil, or garlic. Some delicatessens also sell raspberry and other fruit vinegars. Now go and make that salad dressing!
Think that rice was a white and fluffy but rather bland way of bulking out the good stuff	First change your brand of rice! Buy whole grain basmati or wild rice, then zip up the flavor this way: Heat one teaspoon of olive oil in the saucepan and sauté with one teaspoon of Chinese Five Spice, or Spices for Couscous. Both of these are available at good supermarkets. Now stir in your dry rice, then add the water and do the usual cooking routine. Better?

If You Used to Do This . . .	Now Do This!
Think roast onions tasted like cooked water	Leave small onions whole and slice larger ones in half. Now press two or three whole cloves into each onion and place in the baking pan with potatoes, parsnips, and half the oil you would normally use. Instead, get taste to the max by dissolving a tablespoon of yeast extract in a little warm water and pour over the waiting veg. *Now* roast!

FOOD FACTOR 6: CEREAL FOODS, SNACKS, AND TREATS

Food is one of life's great pleasures, and The Plant Program is not a hair-shirt regime for masochists. I buy sorbets and soy ice creams and organic dairy-free dark chocolate for occasional treats (now that my cancer has gone). Also, I do occasionally eat some of the delicious soups sold in waxed paper cartons now on offer after checking carefully that they contain no dairy products, but I do *not* buy those available in plastic pots (see p. 201).

My favorite treat is fish and chips, which I eat at least once a week now that my cancer has gone, although I remove all the batter unless I buy it from my local fish and chip shop, where they are kind enough to make it without milk. Recently I was struck, walking down a main street in Surrey, by two fast-food shops, one advertising "the great American experience" (cowburgers on white bread) and the other "the great British experience" (fish and chips). If I use fast food, I always choose the British version on health grounds as well as taste.

I eat masses of dried fruit of all descriptions. Prunes contain anticancer chemicals, and figs are an excellent source of calcium. Seeds such as pumpkin, sesame (both a rich source of zinc), and sunflower make delicious snacks and are very nutritious. Traditionally, Chinese people give such seeds and small pieces of fresh or dried fruit to their children as treats rather than sugary sweets, cakes, and cookies, as we tend to do in the West. Until recently the good state of the teeth of most Chinese people clearly reflected this practice.

Much snack food, such as sandwiches and cookies, is based on wheat, which has a bad name with many alternative health practitioners—although I fail to understand why wheat or other gluten-based cereals (barley and rye) are intrinsically bad for people, except where there is clear evidence of a gluten intolerance. (Gluten intolerance, also known as celiac disease, is a genetic disorder that affects between 1 in 150[68] and 1 in 250[69] Americans. Symptoms can include diarrhea, weight loss, and malnutrition.) Most people in developing countries rely on cereals as one of their main sources of food and have traditionally had low levels of the diseases of affluence, including cancer. Wheat consumption is often suggested to be bad because it is linked to settled farming. Barley, oats, maize, and rice, however, were also domesticated from wild cereal grasses at approximately the same time and have been used by farmers for thousands of years, albeit mainly in a labor-intensive, not a capital-intensive, way. Moreover, wheat is generally eaten after it has been processed in some way, whereas rice is traditionally eaten whole. Perhaps the increased incidence of the diseases archaeologists correlate with the beginning of settled farming was due to other factors, including milk consumption and deficiency conditions caused by overexploitation and degradation of land. I do not believe wheat itself to be involved in promoting cancer, although there is some evidence that the herbicide sprays used to eliminate weeds from wheat crops might promote breast cancer. Perhaps wheat is an example of how industrialized agriculture and food production can convert a good, nutrient-rich food into one that many alternative health practitioners feel they must tell us not to eat.

Wheat is now produced mainly by monoculture methods under conditions as prairielike as possible, with hedges bulldozed and biodiversity reduced, so that a high degree of mechanization can be used in the planting and harvesting of crops and the spraying of pesticides. Soil used for such industrialized agriculture becomes exhausted and depleted of essential nutrients because of a lack of animal manure, and these are only partly replaced by inorganic fertilizers.[70] Processing wheat to make white flour for white bread and many commercial pastries removes much of the proteins, vitamins, and minerals, and this residue is often used for animal fodder. To compensate, inorganic nutrients such as chalk as a source of calcium, iron, and vitamins are then added. Despite these additions, such processed flour has often lost much of its bioavailable vitamin B_6, vitamin B_5, and molybdenum, nearly all of its vitamin E, cobalt, and zinc, much of its chromium, and some selenium, too. The degradation of nutritional content is made worse by the addition of bleaches and "improvers" such as potassium bromate, some of which have been shown to be toxic. I always check the list of ingredients carefully when buying bread and ensure that it is free of chemical additives. If I had the time, I would make my own bread with freshly purchased organic wheat or other cereals, using one of the bread-making machines that are now widely available, but my life is far too busy at the moment!

To avoid any potential problems associated with wheat, I use only organic whole wheat brown bread made with stone-ground flour. I eat many other types of organically grown cereals, including oatmeal and oatcakes, organic whole brown rice, and whole wheat brown organic pasta, all widely available in health food stores and increasingly in supermarkets. Despite some recently published versions of anti-breast-cancer diets, there is nothing wrong with muesli providing it is based on organic produce and is not the commercial product made with sugar or milk-derived components. Also, you should use rice, oat, or soy milk or fruit juice rather than dairy milk to moisten it. If you are staying in a hotel, use the juice from fresh fruit salad, or if there is none, use the juice from the prunes that are almost always on the buffet. Fiber is used for the workings of the digestive tract, and according to some alternative health writers it helps to carry excess female hormones such as estrogen out of the system. However, many high-fiber, especially cereal-based, diets contain high levels of a substance known as phytate. This can bind zinc in the digestive tract and make it unavailable for absorption. (Apparently people living on such diets for long periods of time become adapted and can absorb enough zinc and other mineral nutrients to maintain an adequate status, but I think it is important to eat the zinc-containing protein in your diet at least eight hours after eating food such as cereal, which contains high levels of phytates.) Interestingly, the fiber in flaxseed has been shown in experiments not to bind zinc.[71]

INNOCENT INDULGENCES:
Ten Healthy Treats to Keep You Sweet

If You Used to Do This . . .	Now Do This!
Tuck into a giant bag of potato chips while reading the latest novel	Pour a small handful each of sesame, sunflower, and pumpkin seeds into a bowl and munch more nutritiously through your book. Or try roasting the seeds in a pan and sprinkle with soy sauce.
Leave a trail of candy wrappers around the place	Mix your own blend of organic dried fruits such as figs, dates, apricots, mango, and raisins and place little bowls or cartons of them in handy places: the car, your desk, near the phone . . .
Reward yourself with sweet and sticky desserts layered with cream	Take an organic Granny Smith apple, remove the core, and fill it with raisins, chopped banana, cinnamon, and a little maple syrup. Place it in a dish and bake for about 15 minutes. Serve with soy cream or soy ice cream.
Reward yourself with sweet and sticky desserts not layered with cream	Take an organically grown orange, slice it in half, and use a grapefruit knife to slice around the segments. Sprinkle the sliced surface with a tiny pinch of nutmeg or cloves and the merest hint of maple syrup. Bake for about 15 minutes. Serve hot.
Eat whole variety packs of snack crackers in a single sitting	Buy rice cakes and oatcakes and arrange them on a plate with a little hummus, tofu dip, tahini, or homemade salsa.

If You Used to Do This . . .	Now Do This!
Get a sweet craving at least twice a day	Soak a mixture of chopped organic dried fruit in mineral water overnight. When you get your sweet attack, serve a small bowlful dressed with a little rosewater and chopped pumpkin seeds.
Get a serious snack attack once a day	Fight back with a piping hot baked potato heaped with hummus or baked beans. Sometimes a bean salad will do the trick.
Blow out on ice cream and chocolate in any combination	Do it with soy ice cream and dark chocolate instead, or get moderate and serve a homemade chilled fruit soup with a tiny dollop of soy ice cream or soy yogurt.
Eat packaged cookies every day	Pack your own stack of oatcakes spread with jam and made into sandwiches. Sweet, crunchy, and very nutritious.
Eat toast and whatever until the whole loaf was gone	Buy only whole-grain bread made with organic flour and be fussy about what you spread on it. Try tahini, barley miso, mashed banana, or olive pâté.

FOOD FACTOR 7: WHAT TO DRINK

As I mentioned earlier, I drink freshly made vegetable and fruit juices made from organic produce. However, sources of water are more problematic. Before mankind reached the sort of population densities we have now, especially in cities, and before we began to use large quantities of water for washing clothes and cars and power generators and factories, most people would have drunk water from wells, springs, or rivers. Unfortunately, the only way of providing adequate water now is to recycle it by treating or reprocessing water at sewage works. During treatment the water is filtered through progressively finer material to remove particles, microbes, and chemicals, and it is often mixed with other water to dilute harmful chemicals so that their concentration falls below legal requirements. Finally, chlorine is added to kill microbes.

In the early 1990s work by Professor Sumpter at Brunel University in London showed that in several U.K. rivers downstream of sewage works a high proportion (and in some cases 100 percent) of the male fish had been feminized, their testes overgrown with eggs. Some of the chemicals implicated include phthalates from soft plastics, nonyl phenols (breakdown products from detergents and plastics), and residues from birth control or hormone replacement pills. Reprocessed drinking water can contain many other harmful chemicals, including benzene and cancer-causing organic chemicals, pesticides, and disinfection by-products such as trihalomethanes and haloacetic acids. More rigorous limits for disinfection by-products are being legislated for in the United States.[72] For these and other reasons I do not drink water straight from the tap. However, I do not recommend drinking mineral water either, especially from plastic bottles. Moreover, some bottled waters can contain such high levels of radioactivity or nitrates that they would be illegal if they came out of the tap.

I use tap water, but I filter it through charcoal into a glass jug. I have found it impossible to buy a filtration unit made completely of glass, but the plastic is hard and when thoroughly washed is unlikely to release into the water the high concentrations of phthalates associated with soft plastic. After filtering I always boil the water before drinking it to remove or further reduce harmful chemicals and to take out germs not removed by water treatment. These can occur in tap water and bottled water from shallow sources. I always add tea or herbal teas to try to further remove pollutants (lots of organic plant matter absorbs harmful chemicals onto the surface, removing them from the liquid that you drink). This takes out or reduces many harmful chemical residues because they are often large molecules that are hydrophobic—that is, they do not stay in water—and if they are given the opportunity they will attach themselves to something such as charcoal or organic matter instead.

It is particularly important to boil water before drinking when undergoing chemotherapy because the immune system will not be at its best—technically such patients are regarded as immunocompromised instead of immunocompetent (normal with a healthy immune system). Over the past fifteen years or so it has become apparent that a protozoan parasite (called Cryptosporidium), related to the malaria parasite and present in contaminated water supplies, can cause severe sickness, vomiting, dehydration, and diarrhea in immunocompromised people, with symptoms that can persist indefinitely (although the gastroenteritis it causes usually clears up on its own in healthy individuals).

Some of the first diagnosed outbreaks, which occurred because of contamination of the water supply, were in the United States and the United Kingdom; for example, outbreaks in Texas in 1984 and in Ayrshire and Oxfordshire in the late 1980s. In 1993 more than 400,000 people were affected and several people died after Cryptosporidium breached one of Milwaukee, Wisconsin's water filtration plants. Prevention involves boiling (including bottled water if it is from shallow sources) and frequent and thorough hand washing and bedding changes. Infection has been reported in domestic animals, livestock, and wildlife.[73]

I never drink coffee, but I drink lots of Chinese green tea with no milk (if you use lemon, remove the peel first unless you are using unwaxed organic fruits). Extracts of green tea have been shown to prevent cancer in experimental animals, and more recently similar claims have been made about black tea (but I find this more difficult to drink without milk). The chemicals thought to have anticancer properties in green tea are polyphenols known as cathechins, which include epigallo-cathechin-3 gallate, an antioxidant that accounts for much of the solid materials in brewed green tea.[74] It is thought that the well-known anticancer activity of green tea is a result of its inhibiting one of the most frequently overexpressed enzymes in human cancers, called urokinase.[75]

Drinking fluid this way is exactly what the Chinese do. When I first worked in China, I used to wonder what the jam jars with strange-looking bits in the bottom were in the front of taxis. Eventually I realized they were jars of green tea! Chinese, Japanese, and Korean green teas generally contain less pesticide than commonly produced black tea. In China, green tea is valued for its digestive properties and for assisting circulation and regulating body temperature. Preparation of black teas, unlike green teas, involves fermentation.[76] Black tea can contain twice as much caffeine (as theine) as coffee; the tannin content of black tea can also inhibit iron uptake, and brewing black tea oxidizes the cathechins, thus destroying any beneficial effects.[77]

I drink only green tea (or weak black tea without milk or sugar if there is no other choice). I also drink herbal teas, mostly peppermint or chamomile with honey (many people do not like the taste of pure chamomile at first). I also drink fruit teas, but sparingly, because some are so acid that if I drink too much they give me cystitis. Also, some contain chemicals of the kind used to flavor jellies and candies, and I avoid these.

Excess alcohol consumption has long been suggested to be a risk factor for breast cancer. Recent research at the Harvard School of Public Health indicates that the more alcohol women consume, the higher their risk of developing breast cancer, which is increased by up to 40 percent for those drinking three glasses of wine or the equivalent of 30 grams of alcohol a day. The findings, however, were based on studies in the United States, Canada, the Netherlands, and Sweden, countries with some of the highest breast cancer incidences in the world. Certainly alcohol causes problems with the way the liver functions and it has been suggested to increase estrogen and IGF-1 mobilization in the body. Studies are being carried out in Sweden to assess the effects of alcohol on IGF-1 and the proteins that can inactivate IGF-binding proteins.[78] I drank very little alcohol before I had cancer and I had none during treatment. I drink some alcohol now, but keep to real ales, which are rich in nutrients, especially the important B vitamins, and which contain malt and hops which are soothing to the mind and help me to have a good night's sleep. I never drink wine, which is too acid for me and causes me to have cystitis or joint problems. If you must drink wine, have only organically produced wine. Most wine regions produce at least one organic label, and increasingly supermarkets and liquor stores stock these at very reasonable prices. I have seen Chinese men drink alcohol—sometimes lots of it—as beer, rice wine, or *mautai* (distilled rice wine, the equivalent of whisky), but I have rarely seen Chinese women drink alcohol. Chinese men suffer very little with prostate cancer, and I do not believe moderate alcohol consumption to be a primary factor in breast or prostate cancer. If, however, your diet is rich in animal foods containing the hormones and other chemicals that I believe to be the primary factors involved in promoting these types of cancer, alcohol could make matters worse, by increasing levels of circulatin estrogen or free IGF-1, for example.

When I had active cancer I drank no black tea or alcohol and I never drink coffee. One of the benefits of removing these substances from my diet when I was being treated for cancer was that I felt less anxious (without caffeine) and less depressed (without alcohol). Some of my fellow patients who felt the need to drown their sorrows noticeably fared badly, and many were clearly depressed.

THIRST QUENCHERS:
Ten Drinks to Delight You

If You Used to Do This . . .	Now Do This!
Start the day with a hot black one	Make it a hot yannoh instead. This is the finest cereal "coffee" on the market. Try brewing it with 2–3 pods of cardamom and a few whole cloves.
Drink strong tea with milk all day long	If you must have the milky taste, try switching to roibush tea, available at health food stores. It is strong, caffeine-free, and tastes good with soy milk.
Drink black tea with sliced lemon	That's better, but you could try green tea or a strongly flavored herbal tea such as nettle or dandelion.
Treat yourself to a Starbuck's hot chocolate	Order it made with soy milk. When you make it yourself, try making it with carob instead. This is a chocolate-flavored bean that is tasty and nutritious but caffeine-free.

If You Used to Do This . . .	Now Do This!
Guzzle cola all day long	Buy sarsaparilla concentrate from a health food shop or herbalist and dilute to taste with sparkling mineral water.
Swig soft drinks by the gallon	Dilute natural fruit or flower cordials, such as elderflower, with sparkling mineral water. (If you have active breast cancer, prepare freshly made juices.)
Enjoy a jug of iced coffee now and then	Brew the yannoh and cardamom, above, and let it cool. Pour a little into an ice cube tray and freeze. Blend the cooled yannoh with cold soy milk, whisk, and serve with a yannoh ice cube.
Lead a single-handed campaign to double the government recommendations for intake of alcohol	Switch to real beer. Now become a beer historian and expert. Try making your own without a kit. (Your intake will drop, but your enjoyment will soar.)
Spend huge amounts on fresh juices from the refrigerated shelves in the supermarket	Bet you had to shake them first. Make all juices fresh with your own juicer and organic fruit and veg. Try melon, apple and celery, pear, apple and fennel, carrot and parsley, and so on.
Think carrot juice was a cure for sunburn	Make your own with organic carrots. Add a quarter pint of carrot juice to a half pint of cold soy milk, stir well, and serve with a straw.

At a Glance: A Summary of the Main Plant Program Recommendations

Food and Drink I Never Consume

+ Milk: whether organic, whole, skim, semi-skim, or of any other description—from sheep, goats, or cows.
+ Cheese: including so-called vegetarian cheese and cottage cheese.
+ Yogurt: Get the good bacteria from acidophilus capsules from health food shops. But remove gelatin capsules before emptying contents into a glass of soy, rice, oat, or coconut milk or water.
+ Crème fraîche.
+ *Fromage frais.*
+ Cream.
+ Butter.
+ Foods containing any of the above or whey, lactose, milk solids, milk fats, or casein. If in doubt, ask the shop owner or manager and do not allow yourself to be confused—dairy products are dairy products even when they are used in processed or canned foods.
+ Margarine.
+ Beef or pork meat. I also avoid processed meats including pâté because I now follow my mother's practice of not eating anything in which I cannot identify the ingredients.
+ Commercial refined and processed oils prepared using high-pressure or elevated temperatures including unspecified vegetable oils, which may be genetically modified soy or maize oil, canola or rapeseed oil, or products that contain these.
+ Salt, refined white flour or rice, other refined substances such as saccharin, white sugar, or foods containing these products, such as white bread and pasta, which have been chemically altered and depleted of fiber and nutrients.
+ Processed food that comes packaged or in cans, including cookies, cakes, candies, carbohydrates, potato chips, soups, salted nuts, processed meat products such as ham or corned beef, bottled or commercial pickles, canned or cartoned fruit juices, or fruit drinks containing additives or color.
+ Wines, spirits, colored or flavored fizzy drinks.

+ Anything sold in plastic bottles or wrapped in soft plastics (see p. 201).
+ Ready-prepared meals or TV dinners containing gums or starches and emulsifiers to thicken and prevent separation of sauces, and artificial sweeteners, flavorings, or coloring agents.
+ Artificial vitamin or mineral tablets (although I did take selenium combined with vitamins A, C, and E when I had active cancer.

One-Portion-a-Day Food and Drink

These foods are fine as part of a cancer-prevention diet or after recovery, but I did not consume them when I had active cancer.

+ Organically reared chicken or turkey, preferably drumsticks and dark meat.
+ Organically reared duck.
+ Organically reared rabbit.
+ Organically reared lamb.
+ Wild venison or other game.
+ Any fish or shellfish from unpolluted sources including tuna or sea bass and cold water fish such as mackerel, herring, sardines, or wild salmon.
+ Organic eggs from poultry fed on grain.
+ Real ale or cider.

Occasional Treats

Once a week but not when I had active cancer.

+ Fruit sorbet.
+ Soy ice cream.
+ Organic, dairy-free dark chocolate.
+ Fish (but I take off the batter) and chips.
+ Organic bacon.
+ Herbal fruit teas (but not those containing artificial colors or flavorings).
+ Going out for a meal. I choose Thai, Korean, Japanese, and authentic Chinese restaurants; but be aware that some Eastern cuisine avail-

able in the West has been greatly modified to appeal to Westerners. I also go to restaurants of any type that sell truly vegan food.

Food and Drink I Have Lots Of

+ Fruit and dried fruit (organically produced wherever possible).
+ Steamed vegetables (organically produced).
+ Salad vegetables including sprouting seeds, especially bean sprouts and alfalfa.
+ Garlic.
+ Freshly prepared vegetables and fruit juices.
+ Cereals including organic unrefined wheat, oats, barley, and rice, and bread, pasta, and other products made from them.
+ Flavorings made using wine or balsamic vinegar, garlic, herbs such as mint, sage, thyme, coriander, marjoram, and oregano. I use some black pepper, chili, lemongrass, and other spices to make the occasional Eastern dish. I particularly recommend Thai flavorings—remember that Thai people have the lowest breast and prostate cancer mortality rate on record.
+ Nuts and seeds including flaxseed, sunflower, pumpkin, sesame, and spreads such as tahini.
+ Soy including soy milk, tofu, tempeh, miso, and the growing range of organic soy products available; meals such as Jamaican rice and peas—a good meal that provides a good range of proteins.
+ Hummus and taramasalata.
+ Molasses and honey.
+ Green Japanese, Korean, or Chinese teas.
+ Peppermint, chamomile, and nettle herbal teas.
+ Olive oil and other cold-pressed oils such as walnut, pumpkin, or sesame.
+ Organic wine or cider vinegar.

THE STORY OF LIANE BALDOCK

Liane Baldock is a friend of mine who developed breast cancer, follows my diet, and kindly offered to tell her own story.

In June 1996 I sought my GP's advice concerning a small lump on the outside edge of my left breast. He considered it of little significance and claimed there was a three-month wait for appointments at the National Health Service (NHS) specialist breast clinic in my area. He did not feel it was warranted to refer me to it. I requested a second opinion and was referred to a private senior general surgeon in July. I was told by him: "If ever you have breast cancer it will have nothing to do with this lump." I requested a needle biopsy to be sure, but was told it was too small to locate accurately. I was not informed (and did not know myself) about ultrasound scans at that stage. By November the lump was easily visible when my arm was raised and in December I returned to request the surgeon to remove it privately to avoid another long wait on the NHS, as it still "could not be considered an emergency." Two days later he removed it under a local anesthetic, and as I slid down off the table he said, "I'd be willing to bet a million pounds this biopsy comes back negative." Pity I did not take him up on it! Ten days later I returned to have the stitches removed and to be told (by his nurse!) that it was malignant and that I would need further surgery. Finally I was put under the care of a specialist NHS breast surgeon, who pulled out all the stops for me, seeing me within two days and operating himself the following week.

I was deeply shocked and particularly devastated partly because my attempts to do all the right things had not resulted in the early diagnosis I knew to be so important and because my GP and the general surgeon had continually assured me that it was not breast cancer. Neither took it seriously or seemed concerned.

Jane was one of the first people I turned to for advice and support. I had been told to come off hormone replacement therapy at once, and I also gave up all dairy products immediately. I had known about her theories for several years and the research she had done seemed to make sense. I had admired her attitude to her own more serious problems and her scientific approach to alternative therapies that are not yet accepted by the U.K. medical establishment. At the very least it was something positive I could do to help myself, while the specialist medics took over my life for the next three months with a lumpectomy and lymph removal, followed by radiation therapy.

Thankfully no chemotherapy was necessary, as my lymph glands were clear. I refused to take tamoxifen—to the obvious annoyance of my oncologist. She seemed to want to put everyone on it indiscriminately, without ever going into the rest of their medical history. I had had abnormal uterine cells a year or so before and did know that tamoxifen might increase the risk of cancer of the uterus.

As I work at a university I had access to medical research papers and obtained a couple mentioned by the Bristol Cancer Centre on work done in Scandinavia.[79] From that research it appeared that high daily doses of co-enzyme Q_{10} seemed to make breast tumors regress. This has been totally dismissed by the British cancer research teams I have tried to discuss it with. Nevertheless I have been taking it now for three years.

I feel that, at this still relatively early stage (only three and a half years since diagnosis), it would be tempting fate to say any more, but now I have at last got over the effects of the radiation therapy, which left me with what can only be described as crushing exhaustion for almost two years, I do feel pretty fit, although still very wary and on the alert for any potential problem. I also feel that I am doing all I can to reduce the risk of a recurrence by eating a much healthier diet. This includes far more fruit, vegetables, and fish, less saturated fats, and no dairy products—except for the odd cheese sandwich, which I find irresistible at times and which is the only thing I really miss!

If substituting (genetic-modification-free!) soy-based or vegetable oil products for dairy products helps to reduce the incidence or recurrence of breast cancer, it is certainly worth it and no great hardship, compared with the alternative.

6.

The Plant Program—
The Lifestyle Factors

There are important things apart from diet that you can change to help cut your risk of breast and prostate cancer. In this chapter I explain why you should make these changes and how to do so successfully: from coping strategies for stress to ways of avoiding harmful substances in your environment.

As well as dietary factors there are lifestyle factors we can change to cut our risk of developing breast cancer. These range from the way we buy and store our food to the way we cope with stress. Here I will take you through the five most important lifestyle factors.

LIFESTYLE FACTOR 1: VITAMIN AND MINERAL SUPPLEMENTS

In general I prefer to eat whole foods because, as I have indicated, problems often arise when we try to separate food into constituent parts. Moreover, vitamin/mineral pills are often synthesized from coal or petroleum derivatives. Also, taking too much of one or another man-made supplement can cause a deficiency elsewhere in our diet. For example, taking the trace element molybdenum blocks copper intake. The body knows how to deal with nutrients from natural foods but may absorb too much or too little from man-made chemical supplements. Hence I take no man-made vitamin or mineral pills, although for the six months when I was undergoing chemotherapy I took tablets that combined selenium with vitamins A, C, and E.

Selenium status can be marginal to deficient in some U.S. diets, and it is important for immune function generally and as an antioxidant. This trace mineral is essential to health, though only required in minute quantities. In the United States, the National Research Council has recommended a daily intake of 50 to 200 mcg of selenium for adults (a microgram is one thousandth of a milligram, so 200 mcg equal 0.2 mg). However, one authority—Gerhard Schrauzer, Ph.D., of the University of California—says that 250 to 300 mcg can protect against most cancers and that most people consume only about 100 mcg daily.[1] At higher doses, selenium can be highly toxic to the human body. Although it is not certain at precisely what level selenium begins to cause adverse effects, it has been found that high doses including too many or too potent selenium tablets per day can make hair and nails fall out and can affect the nervous system.[2]

Selenium works best in conjunction with vitamin E, since both are antioxidants and can increase the production of antibodies by up to thirty times,[3] thereby greatly enhancing your immune response. Together they help to detoxify your body and prevent the formation of free radicals. Selenium is naturally present in the soil, and the quantities available in our food relate to soil levels of selenium where the food was grown.[4] A study of the health effects of selenium compared its distribution in soil across the United States with a map detailing the national cancer rates. It was found that those areas with high levels of cancer corresponded with places having low levels of selenium in the soil.[5]

A study undertaken at the University of Tampere, Finland, involved taking blood samples from 21,172 Finnish men. The samples were then frozen. Eleven years after the samples had been taken, 143 men had contracted lung cancer. The researchers found that the men who eventually developed lung cancer had less selenium in their blood than those who did not. Overall, it was found that people with the lowest selenium levels were 3.3 times more likely to develop lung cancer than those with high levels. The researchers said their results were "in accord with other studies which strongly suggest that poor selenium nutrition is a highly significant risk factor for lung cancer."[6]

In West Germany, a study conducted at the University of Bonn has shown that selenium can protect against the harmful effects of ultraviolet radiation. Blood selenium levels were examined in 101 patients with malignant melanoma (a lethal form of skin cancer) and compared with those in a control group of healthy people. The skin cancer patients showed a significantly lower level of selenium, and the researchers concluded that their results "strongly suggest that sub-optimal selenium nutrition preceded the onset of the disease and may even have contributed to its genesis."[7]

Industrialized agriculture and food production may well be leading to subclinical deficiencies in vitamins and minerals. Also, obesity can cause deficiency conditions. I am not overweight and I rely on a varied diet of organically produced food to provide most of my needs. If I feel I need extra vitamins and minerals I use freshly made organic juices, which are less likely than pill supplements to cause toxicity or imbalances. I do, however, take kelp to avoid iodine deficiency and also brewer's yeast, which is a good source of many trace elements—including iron, zinc, selenium, and chromium (which is protective against diabetes)—and B vitamins, which are important if the body is to synthesize important compounds such as co-enzyme Q_{10}. Co-enzyme Q_{10} has been shown to be essential to the optimal functioning of all cell types, and there is evidence that supplementation with co-enzyme Q_{10} helps regression of breast cancer.[8] Co-enzyme Q_{10} is also an antioxidant and free radical scavenger. The body is capable of synthesizing adequate quantities given a good diet, especially one rich in the B vitamins and minerals concentrated in brewer's yeast. Also, soy contains co-enzyme Q_{10}.

Siberian ginseng and parnox or true ginseng are both reputed to help immunity and to overcome tiredness and debility associated with cancer treatment including radiation therapy (although the Bristol diet recommends against them). I use only whole roots or root pieces of ginseng, not teas or extracts. I used them occasionally, especially toward the end of my radiation therapy treatment. They are available from Eastern shops and some good health stores.

Food Supplements I Use
Brewer's yeast (six tablets a day), red clover (a quarter of a teaspoon a day), Icelandic kelp (six tablets a day).* These are all natural and not synthetic substances. I took tablets containing selenium and vitamins A, C, and E when I had active cancer.

LIFESTYLE FACTOR 2: FOOD PACKAGING

Food packaging is very important. A recent report on the abundance of chemicals that mimic the female hormone estrogen from the authoritative British Institute of Environment and Health (IEH) has suggested that a group of chemicals called phthalates seriously disrupt reproduction in animals (including damaging the testes in males). Scientific experiments suggest that certain phthalates may cause birth defects, cancer, testicular atrophy, and sterility.[9] One of the main sources of phthalates identified in the IEH report was soft plastics such as those which may come into contact with food. The chemicals leak from the plastic into the food and then accumulate in our body fat (remember, a considerable proportion of breast tissue is fat). Try whenever possible to buy food in good old-fashioned brown paper bags—be prepared to make a fuss if necessary. One of my friends dumps all plastic wrappings at supermarket checkout counters, although I must say I have never dared go so far as that. If you find it impossible to buy food not prepacked in plastic, and this is increasingly difficult, try to wash food as thoroughly as possible or, in the case of vegetables, peel or scrape off the surface that has been most in contact with the plastic. Unfortunately, the chemicals concerned are fat-soluble, so it is best to avoid them if possible, since they are difficult to remove by washing.

---

*The actual quantity of tablets or clover depends on the brand. Be sure to read the instructions on the package and follow them closely.

LIFESTYLE FACTOR 3: COOKING

Love it or hate it, cooking is an essential part of our diet and lifestyle. In among all the aromas and sizzles, it has an effect on the food that can be enhancing or potentially destructive. For instance, it changes starches, proteins, and some vitamins into forms that the body can absorb readily. It also releases nutrients that are otherwise unavailable in some foods—like the amino acid tryptophan in cornmeal. Cooking of some foods is necessary to destroy toxic substances, such as those found in red beans, and cooking also makes some foods, like meat, palatable. However, cooking can destroy and leach out fragile nutrients in food, although there are ways you can reduce this nutrient loss.

I lightly steam vegetables in a stainless-steel or bamboo steamer. Otherwise I stir-fry lightly after first thoroughly washing and dipping vegetables in boiling water as the Chinese do. Fruit and vegetables should be eaten as raw as possible in order to preserve the vitamins and enzymes they contain. Recent research, for example, suggests that cooking broccoli destroys the anticancer chemical that it contains. I use only organic extra-virgin olive oil to soften or gently fry vegetables. Any meat I eat is cooked slowly in the oven or under a broiler, and the fish I eat is just lightly broiled. I add no additional fat or salt to meat or fish, which I cook slowly with herbs or garlic and occasionally black pepper or other spices for flavoring. I do not own a microwave and try to avoid food cooked or heated in one. Unlike normal heating, microwaving works by vibrating the water molecules in food. This generates free radicals and I suspect would not destroy as many "bad" chemicals as ordinary cooking (although I have been unable to find any data on this). Apart from anything else, I do not like the taste of microwaved food. There is no comparison between the taste of a baked potato cooked in the traditional way and the soggy, unpleasant-tasting equivalent prepared by microwaving. Here are some general guidelines:

+ If you cook with fat, don't let it become so hot that it starts to smoke. At this temperature the essential fatty acid linoleic acid is destroyed.

+ Fats that have been used for cooking once should be discarded, since the linoleic acid and vitamins A and C will have been lost; they may also have become oxidized and rancid and hence potentially carcinogenic.

+ If you boil food, do so for the minimum amount of time and then use the water for stock afterward. The fragile water-soluble vitamins as well as some minerals leach into cooking water, which is why soups are so nutritious.

+ Don't add bicarbonate of soda to cooking water, even if you see it recommended in cookbooks for cooking beans, peas, or lentils. It destroys valuable B vitamins.

+ Prepare food immediately before cooking—remember that vitamin C is destroyed once cells are damaged in vegetables—and for the same reason try not to chop them too fine. Scrubbing vegetables is better than peeling them.

+ Once prepared, immerse the vegetables in ready boiling water straight away.

+ Use pans with close-fitting lids and avoid using copper pans, which encourage oxidation and vitamin C loss. I use stainless-steel pans and bamboo baskets for steaming.

+ Once food is cooked, eat it right away. Keeping it warm will only result in further nutrient loss, which is why eating out too frequently may be less than healthy for you.

LIFESTYLE FACTOR 4: DEALING WITH STRESS

The idea that cancer could be cured by thinking positively had always seemed ill founded to me. I certainly did not believe that I could be cured of breast cancer simply by thinking positively. One of the particular problems with the "think positive" approach is that people who do not get better often feel guilty that they are not trying hard enough. Sometimes this is reinforced by their friends, and the patients become convinced that they remain ill simply because they are not being positive enough. In the book *You Can Heal Your Life* by Louise Hay, there is a list of diseases and their probable causes. In the case of cancer (all types presumably), the probable cause is given as "deep hurt, long-standing resentment, deep secret or grief eating away at the self; carrying hatreds; what's the use." The advice is to develop a new thought pattern as follows: "I lovingly forgive and release all of the past. I choose to fill my world with joy. I love and approve of myself." Fine, but I prefer a more rational approach, which seeks to remove cancer-causing chemicals from my life.

It has also been claimed that there is a particular personality type that is likely to be affected by breast cancer. Much has been written about the "cancer personality," especially by Lawrence LeShan, an American psychotherapist who worked with over 200 cancer patients. According to LeShan, the typical personality had an emotionally deprived youth, followed in later life by a period of fulfillment in an intense relationship or through all-involving work, followed by the loss of that relationship or work, at which time the cancer occurs. The other main characteristic is the person's inability to express anger, particularly in his/her own defense; such a person is often described by others as being like a saint. LeShan believed that this pattern fitted 76 percent of his patients. This is certainly not a description of me or my life, and I cannot think of anyone else I know who has had breast cancer who fits this description!

All carefully controlled research indicates that this theory is wrong. The concept is unhelpful and again tends to lead to feelings of guilt. As indicated earlier, the problem is one of chemistry and is rooted in the Western diet. The book *Wild Swans* by Jung Chang provides a vivid example of the high levels of stress that Chinese women have suffered in the past, yet they maintain low breast cancer rates except when they have changed to a Western diet.

Because stress has been implicated as an important factor in breast cancer, people can become worried and hence more stressed by problems so that a vicious circle is set up. When I was ill with cancer I found that as soon as a stressful situation arose I became so worried that the stress would cause my illness to return that my distress about situations increased rather than decreased. Over the last six and a half years I have faced up to some extremely stressful situations in my family life and at work, and yet my cancer has not returned—because fundamentally it was a problem caused by harmful chemicals from my food and the environment causing problems in my body. Now that my diet and lifestyle are sound, I cope very well with stress.

However, for your health and general well-being it is helpful to reduce the stress and distress in your life as much as possible, and there *is* scientific evidence that stress has physiological effects, suggesting that it is worthwhile working on methods of reducing or removing sources of stress. Folklore and old wives' tales are sometimes based on observation and wisdom passed down from one generation to the next. At the time I was ill I remembered some of the earthy old ladies in the village I grew up in who used to talk about situations "worrying their tits off." I wondered whether there could be some basis for this expression! The chemical changes caused by stress would need another whole book to describe. Hormones from the adrenal gland secreted as part of the body's "fight or flight" mechanism increase the amount of blood sugar available, boost heart rate, and slow down digestive function to enable us to run or fight. Too much for too long, however, affects the immune system.

When humans are confronted by an important loss or change in their life—such as a diagnosis of breast cancer—their emotions are likely to follow a pattern that is well known to counselors and others trained to help with our emotional well-being. Initially, shock and numbness may be experienced, followed by resistance, gradual acceptance, and depression before beginning to let go of the old reality and adjust to the new one. People differ in the intensity of their emotions and the time taken for each part of the cycle. Indeed, in the case of cancer, some people simply give up hope and never leave the "trough of despair."

In my case, when confronted with problems I tend to move to the "what can be done about it?" stage very quickly, and of course one of the frustrations with being confronted by a diagnosis of breast cancer is that according to orthodox medicine the answer is "nothing." If you have heart disease you can follow a diet and exercise plan; if you have an infectious illness you can take tablets and rest; but with breast cancer you are told there is nothing you can do. The conventional risk factors, which we have already discussed, translate into this: it is too late and there was little or nothing you could have done to prevent breast cancer anyway.

As I have explained earlier in the book, *there is a lot you can do to help yourself* through changes in diet and lifestyle that are crucially important. The diet in itself, in addition to helping you fight cancer directly, will help your state of mental and emotional well-being by providing a better balance of the essential nutrients (including zinc, iodine, B vitamins, and the essential fatty acids) your brain needs.

Dealing with the Stress of Breast Cancer

Let us look at some of the emotional problems associated with coping with breast cancer. A large percentage of people become depressed, especially after losing a breast. In a study at three cancer centers, 47 percent of those diagnosed with cancer had a level of distress equivalent to that seen in a true psychiatric disorder.[10] One of the things I was very worried about, and I think most women who have had a mastectomy are, is how different people will react to you. Will you become an object of pity or will people make jokes about you? I was particularly worried about going back to work, especially in such a male-dominated office. In fact, everyone was incredibly kind, sensitive, and considerate. Indeed, one of my colleagues who had been one of my fiercest opponents professionally was one of the first to write to me. Dr. Peter Allen, at the time BGS's chief geologist, sent me a long, carefully thought out, sensitive letter that actually anticipated and addressed all my worst fears. He set out clearly and unequivocally how much everyone valued me as a person and as a scientist and how I should not worry too much about my physical appearance: whatever happened, my colleagues' feelings and respect for me would not change. It was a truly wonderful letter, which I shall always keep with my most treasured mementos. Peter and I still enjoy our professional spats, but I count him and his wife, Joyce, among my dearest friends.

Some marriages and family relationships break down following the wife and mother's suffering from breast cancer. Moreover, many women who have developed breast cancer have done so after trying to come to terms with distressing situations in their lives such as the breakdown of their marriage. I shall try to share with you some of the coping strategies I developed with the help of a wonderful psychotherapist whose help was made available to me by Charing Cross Hospital. It was difficult for me to agree to see her initially because of fear evoked by my childhood memories of the appalling treatment my father had received at the hands of psychiatrists, combined with difficult experiences with my first husband, also a psychiatrist. When I expressed my reservations to her, she quickly reassured me. She had trained initially as a surgeon at Cambridge University before becoming a psychiatrist and finally a psychotherapist. She specialized in helping people who have had limbs amputated come to terms with their problems. She assured me that she would not under any circumstances suggest the use of ECT or drugs.

With the help of my psychotherapist I was able to come to terms with the loss of my breast. Also she helped me to address and come to terms with problems in my life and personality and reactions. I learned that unresolved feelings of fear, anger, and guilt are especially damaging, negative emotions. With her help, I revisited, reinterpreted, and finally dealt with events in my past and memories that generated negative emotions. In some cases I wrote to or telephoned people I had not spoken to for years to try to heal unpleasant situations and reduce my emotional baggage. But in some situations this was not possible and the only way to come to terms with the past was to develop a new perspective.

I will give one example of how I learned to turn an extremely negative situation into something positive. Like many first marriages, mine ended in a breakup: in my case, a particularly unpleasant and protracted process that caused me an enormous amount of personal grief and anxiety. My father was ill at the time and my mother was working hard to keep both of them. With no family support of my own I was persuaded to allow my former parents-in-law to care for my son on the basis that my ex-husband and I would stay friends and when our futures were more settled we could decide what was in our son's best interest.

It emerged at the time of the custody hearing that my son had been staying with my ex-husband a great deal, so the court took the view that he should remain in the situation with which he was familiar, and I was merely granted access. An awkward, and awful, situation; and for me, the saddest part has been the almost total lack of contact between me and my son. With my psychotherapist's help, I eventually managed to understand how this situation came about. As I came to understand what had happened, I became more determined than ever that I would survive. I decided that whenever my son feels able to come back to me, I shall be there for him—a strong and worthwhile person who loves him dearly. In this way, I learned to turn a terrible situation of chronic stress full of hurt and anger into a reason to survive. With help, we can do the same with even the most distressing situations. I found psychotherapy helpful even over the few months I worked with my doctor. According to MIND, the mental health charity, psychotherapy may last for several years and is particularly helpful in understanding and coming to terms with past events.

With my psychotherapist's help I learned two other coping strategies that I found particularly helpful in dealing with cancer. The first is cognitive therapy. Part of being a creative thinker, which I need to be as a scientist, is that I develop large "worry castles" from one or two odd bricks. In dealing with cancer it is particularly easy to develop frightening scenarios for the future. Cognitive therapy teaches you to trace the building of the worry castle backward and stop at the facts. You can then develop a more sensible, rational, less frightening vision. Again according to MIND, cognitive therapy is about learning to think and behave in positive ways. It is a type of behavioral therapy that is helpful in overcoming negative thinking. My psychotherapist also taught me how to be more assertive without being aggressive, which helps avoid situations where one is affected by negative emotions. For example, if you calmly but clearly state your concerns or dislikes, many situations that lead to negative emotions can be avoided. There are many excellent books on cognitive therapy and assertive behavior, which are well worth reading.

I have to say that I found counseling of the type based on trying to release any pent-up emotions far less helpful than the psychotherapy sessions, which were intellectual and analytical and gave me new understanding and insights into situations so that I could develop clear, simple coping strategies. The analogy I would use about my counseling sessions is that of a pond in which emotions had settled to the bottom and the water had cleared, and every week I was encouraged to put in a large stick and stir it around until I became upset. Also, some counselors are trained never to give reassurance, and I found that by repeating answers to "How do you feel about that?" or "What is your worst fear?" I was giving my brain only negative feedback and reinforcing my fears. Others I know have found counseling very helpful—it just did not work well for me. I also tried self-help and support groups but found that these made me feel I was "wallowing in breast cancer" and I found them depressing. Again, others I know have found attending such groups helpful.

The person I found most helpful was a lady who has become one of my dearest friends—Peggy Heason, who is a trained hypnotherapist. For one thing, having brought up three children in the war, cared for six years for a husband with a stroke, and helped see her four grandchildren through school and into university, she has huge funds of common sense and she was prepared to reassure me where she could. But above all, she was always there for me. She cared for me, but she was not so emotionally involved as my own mother, husband, or children, so she was better able to help me. If you have breast cancer or any other serious problems in your life, my advice is to find yourself a Peggy Heason. I went to relaxation sessions with her and I also used her relaxation tape a great deal.[11]

The basis of most techniques for reducing stress and tension is relaxation. First turn off the telephone, doorbell, etc. so you will not be interrupted. Then turn off the light or draw the curtains and lie flat (I do this without a pillow—at most use only one) and make sure you are warm and comfortable. Then systematically relax each part of your body beginning with your toes, then your feet, your lower legs, gradually progressing up through the body. Repeat until you feel totally relaxed. This way you relax each bit of you from toe to top. There are several good relaxation tapes based on these methods, but Peggy Heason's was the one that I found the best. At the same time I used diaphragm breathing, which is very relaxing. When we are anxious we tend to take lots of shallow breaths, using only our rib cage. Diaphragm breathing is a technique to ensure that you are using your full lung capacity by using the large muscle called the diaphragm at the base of the lung cavity to suck in and expel air. You simply place your hands on your abdomen and make sure that they go up and down as you breathe in and out. Used with imagery, you can accompany your relaxation by imagining yourself walking through a beautiful calm garden listening to the birdsong or walking along a beautiful beach with waves gently crashing on the sand. It is possible to buy tapes to guide you through imagery and relaxation, but do listen to them first; do not rely simply on the promotional statement. I found some voices on tapes that I bought without first listening incredibly irritating. It is important to find ones that you enjoy and find helpful because you will probably use them many times. Many such tapes are readily available from health and new age shops. Some include affirmations (quiet verbal instructions) and subliminal messages to your body. I also learned a technique of meditation that I still use, and despite being such a simple method, it clears worries out of the mind and allows deep relaxation. I chose the words *candle* and *crystal* and I repeat one of them continuously in my mind as I visualize the candle gently flickering or the crystal sparkling. After a time I feel truly relaxed. I found meditation difficult at first because I am normally a busy-busy sort of person, but the technique really does clear my mind and helps me in my work, especially in solving problems. I think yoga would also be helpful, although I did not use it. There is a great deal of evidence of the effectiveness of such techniques in reducing stress and tension and the physical symptoms that stress creates in the body; for example, several of the methods described lower blood pressure.

Another technique sometimes used for cancer patients is visualization. Visualization involves imagining your body killing the cancer and removing the debris from your body, and finally visualizing situations where you are well and whole again. The visualization technique was made famous by the Simontons in the United States. It typically involves going into visions of cancer being attacked and cleaned up by the body's defense system. This is how one of the visions begins: "Your white blood cells are fish swimming in and eating up the grayish cancer cells. Project this image as if it were on a screen that you're viewing in your mind's eye. When you have that image very clearly, then *become* one of the fish and lead the rest of the pack into the attack. Feel yourself as the fish eating. At the end of each visualization, imagine yourself engaging in activities you would pursue if you were healthy. Picture yourself at the healthiest time in your life and create images of the present, feeling just that way." I found visualization techniques unhelpful, but others feel better for using them.

So far I have not said much about my husband, my children, or my mother. Perhaps this is because at the time we were all so distressed that we coped badly as a family. My mother was an elderly widow living alone and I am her only child. With Dr. John Camac's help I worked hard to shield her from the worst of the situation. John and her local vicar gave her tremendous support and she found great comfort in her Christianity. At all times I told my husband the truth and also told my daughter, Emma, as kindly and unfrighteningly as possible when the cancer kept coming back in 1993. I was also "gently truthful" with Tom, my youngest son. At the time, my husband was working in Nottingham looking after Tom while I was treated in London. Hence he was hardly ever able to attend clinics or treatment sessions with me, and he often found it difficult to talk about my illness. Peter would help me a lot with housework and shopping and other practical tasks, but he found it difficult to talk about emotions. At the time I was very resentful about this. I blamed it on his stiff-upper-lip upbringing at public school and Cambridge. However, having discussed those feelings with Peter since, I realize that his reactions were not because he did not care but because he cared too much. He found the situation extremely upsetting, especially seeing me undergoing chemotherapy. In order to avoid letting me see his distress he preferred not to become involved in discussions because he thought he would break down in front of me.

I began writing this book partly for young women like my daughter, Emma. She was deeply distressed from the time I first developed cancer when she was 13 until I recovered when she was 19. She is an extremely clever and capable young woman who had always been good at her schoolwork, especially mathematics and science. Shortly before my illness she was one of a few children chosen to represent physics at an evening designed to impress the parents of prospective students at her school. Unfortunately, my illness affected her studies, and for a long time she appeared to be an angry young woman. Only recently have I come to understand what she went through and how much she suffered because of my illness. When I first became ill in 1987 she had only recently developed breasts herself, and there was her mother with a deadly disease in her breasts, which it seemed might kill her. Previously Emma had seen me only as someone totally in control, someone who could always explain things, put things right, make things better—probably more than most of her friends' mothers. Certainly she would bring lots of her little friends' problems to me. Suddenly I was transformed from being a secure pillar in her life to being a victim of something against which I appeared to be helpless in defending myself. Emma is strong and courageous and has worked hard to recover her life, to "get back on track," and now has a very successful career as an account manager with a dynamic young advertising and marketing company in London. We are totally devoted to each other. Only recently, when we went on a "shop 'til you drop" trip together, did I notice how often she spontaneously hugged me or put her arm through mine. She sometimes talks in front of me now about how frightened she was that she would lose me. Emma has helped me to write this book by providing information, encouragement, and support.

Tom, my younger son, was 6 when I was first diagnosed with breast cancer and did not understand what was happening at the time. In 1993, when I had recurrences of breast cancer four times in seven months, he was 11, and like Emma, his schoolwork also suffered for a time. Nevertheless, he was very supportive emotionally. He was able to help me a great deal without showing his own distress. We were able to talk about this situation a lot, and he helped to heal problems that developed between the rest of us. He will be studying medicine at Cambridge. I know he will be a wonderful doctor.

What I learned was how important it is to understand how distressed your family is, if your relationships are to survive cancer. They will all react differently. They are having to come to terms with their own distress, fears, and anxieties about your illness as well as helping and supporting you. They have different personalities with different capabilities and methods of coping. I soon learned not to dump my fears, feelings, and anxieties onto them—they were too close and too frightened and upset already, and as a family we could quickly enter damaging downward-spiraling emotional situations.

I learned instead to rely on others who cared about me but who were not so close that their fears became amplified and spiraled out of control. I found my women friends, my vicar Julian Reindorp, my former doctor John Camac, and Peggy Heason, whom I have already mentioned, the best equipped to help me. They knew me well enough to care about me and give me support, but there was not the intense emotion that there is in the family. A group of my women friends, all professionals with busy lives, each gave some of their time to take me to the hospital and stay with me during radiation therapy and chemotherapy treatments. Somehow they worked together as an efficient team, each giving the help they could and the time they could spare, to provide me with a wonderful cocoon of total care. When they asked me how they could help, I managed to shed my typically British reserve and independence and tell them.

Working with your friends is a two-way process and can be very helpful. If you want to do something for a friend with cancer, ask sincerely how you can help and show that you mean it. All sorts of practical things—helping collect children, doing some shopping, going with them for treatment—mean so much at such times. Here's how friends in London helped me (in addition to coming to Charing Cross on several occasions for treatment sessions with me). Edna Lewis, an architect with her own practice and my neighbor in London, was always there for me, often just listening to my fears in her quiet way or getting help for me from my local vicar, Julian Reindorp. While my husband was away in China the fifth and last time my cancer came back, she slept at my house and manned the telephone. She also helped by talking to Emma and Tom a lot and being there for them. Vicky Guiton, a talented interior designer with her own business, helped me in many ways, from tidying up my kitchen to coming with me to ensure that my unnecessary wig looked good after my hairdresser had restyled it. She introduced two of her other friends to me to help provide support—one of them, Sarah Scott, a retired social worker, was like Vicky herself, a tower of strength. Roberta Stoker, a talented artist, and Choo Simmonds, a mathematics lecturer, made lots of visits and endlessly supported me, often doing shopping for me. Iris Campbell, a brilliant children's fashion designer, kept me endlessly supplied with organic vegetables from her own garden and was a port in a storm for Tom whenever he was in London. Jenny Long and Maria Calvert also made lots of visits, took me out, and gave me masses of support and encouragement. Sarah Wherry, now a senior publisher, took me out a lot, was a second mum to Emma, and when I was at my lowest ebb with the big lump in my neck, forced me to buy myself a new shirt. I still have it. Sarah now agrees that she bullied me into making some gesture to show myself I still had a future at a time when I had virtually given up any hope of surviving. Other friends in Nottingham, especially Penny Tutty, gave me lots of practical help by caring for Tom—often having him to stay with her family for days at a time.

Some friends could not cope—they did not visit or telephone and distanced themselves until I recovered. This is a common experience for cancer patients. You should try to understand that these people do care about you, they just do not know how to cope themselves. You should not allow yourself to become bitter. Let them back into your life when they feel able to come. When I was ill I found on occasion that I simply could not talk to anyone who had any connection with cancer, let alone breast cancer sufferers. My mind was telling me that I could not take any more, but it certainly was not because I did not care. I just had to let go. On one occasion while I was having lunch with a group of friends at work, someone started talking about a colleague whose wife had cancer, thinking, I suppose, that I would be able to offer help. Instead of helping or offering advice, I made some excuse and rushed out of the room. All the people there later told me that they understood. (Since 1994, when I first began to realize that my cancer had gone, I have been able to advise other cancer sufferers or their friends who have asked for my help.)

During my illness, I found it helpful to keep working and took the minimum of sick leave—for example, four days twice a month when I was on chemotherapy (two days for treatment and the following days to recover from the nausea). This gave me a sense of purpose and took my mind off my problems. Many other friends and colleagues with cancer or with partners with cancer have also found the routine of going to work helpful in coping with the disease. Of course, this depends on the type of work you do, the working environment, and your personality, and it requires a supportive boss and colleagues. The head of BGS at the time, Dr. Peter Cook, and his wife, Norma, were wonderful to me, often telephoning and arranging dinner parties to cheer me up. Dr. David Morgan, my deputy at the time, went out of his way to ensure that I felt involved in decision making. He refused to move into my office but sat there for several hours a day doing my work on the days I was away for treatment. I had left lots of high-heeled shoes under my desk, and apparently he put up with much teasing about stepping into my shoes rather than ask me or my husband to move them, because he thought this might upset me. We also have a wonderful Welfare Officer at BGS, the Reverend Howard Bateson, a former geologist and now a canon, who was immensely supportive and kind. Hilary Heason, BGS's press officer, and my then secretary, Janet Drury, provided female support in my male-dominated workplace. Friends and colleagues showered me with flowers, messages, and cards, and they telephoned me a lot—this was very important in maintaining my morale. At the time I thought the situation was reminiscent of the story of Peter Pan, where everyone has to clap their hands if they wish Tinkerbell to recover her health. If you have a friend with cancer, do whatever you can—even if you only send a card. The whole episode was a great learning experience for me. Previously I had been highly competitive and ambitious, and people and relationships had come second, third, or fourth in my list of priorities. Learning to let people into my life made me a much better and happier person and, amazingly, also much more successful!

I think that the best way of coping with cancer emotionally can be summed up by quoting a friend and colleague, Dr. Chris Evans, whose wife, Norma, sadly died of cancer in 1995: "I learned during the four years that Norma was ill that we all react differently. There is no right or wrong way. There are people out there who can help and people who are going through the same thing. These people can suggest a range of coping strategies, but friendship, openness, and love are at the heart of most."

The Big Dos and Don'ts

+ Do not believe the old adage "cancer equals death." Today, many cancers are curable; others can be controlled for long periods during which new treatments may become available.
+ Do not believe that you caused your cancer. There is no evidence linking specific personalities, emotional states, or painful life events to the development of cancer.
+ Do rely on strategies that helped you solve problems in the past, such as gathering information, talking to others, and finding ways to feel in control. Seek help if they don't work.
+ Do not feel guilty if you can't keep a "positive" attitude all the time. Low periods will occur, no matter how good you are at coping. There is no evidence that these periods have a negative effect on your health. If they become too frequent or severe, though, seek help.
+ Do use support and self-help groups if they make you feel better. Leave any that make you feel worse.
+ Do not be embarrassed to seek counsel from a mental-health professional. It is a sign of strength, not weakness, and it may help you tolerate your symptoms and treatments better.
+ Do use any methods that aid you in gaining control over your emotions, such as meditation and relaxation.
+ Do find a doctor of whom you can ask questions and with whom you feel mutual respect and trust. Insist on being a partner with him/her in your treatment. Ask what side effects to expect and be prepared for them. Anticipating problems often makes them easier to handle if they occur.

✦ Do not keep your worries to yourself. If the person closest to you can cope, involve him/her. If your partner finds it difficult, you may need to involve a group of friends so that each can give you some support. If all else fails, phone a local befrienders or Samaritan group (befrienders.org) and talk to them of your fears. Ask a close friend to accompany you on visits to the doctor when treatments are to be discussed. Research shows that you often don't hear or absorb information when you are very anxious; a second person will help you interpret what was said.

✦ Do explore spiritual and religious beliefs and practices that may have helped you in the past. They may comfort you and even help you find meaning in the experience of illness.

✦ Do not abandon your treatment in favor of an alternative method, especially those that make no sense and are irrational. But do change your diet and lifestyle in the ways described here to help overcome your disease and withstand treatment.[12]

LIFESTYLE FACTOR 5: AVOIDING HARMFUL SUBSTANCES IN YOUR ENVIRONMENT

Cancer cells are relatively big, and when they spread they usually get trapped in the first network of capillaries—the very fine blood vessels that take blood to and from all the tissues in our bodies—that they encounter downstream of their origin. The first highly vascularized organ encountered by blood leaving most organs in our bodies is the lung. The intestine is an exception—from there the blood supply goes to the liver first. Hence in the case of all types of cancer, the organs to protect from secondary tumors as much as possible are the lungs and liver. This is particularly important in the case of breast cancer. I therefore decided to cut my exposure to all cancer-causing and potentially cancer-causing chemicals as much as possible.

The effects of exposure to harmful chemicals depend on the dose, the duration, how you are exposed, and the presence of other chemicals. The main task of the lungs is to exchange "old blood" containing carbon dioxide created by body processes for "new blood" invigorated with fresh oxygen. They can cope with some dust, particles, and bad chemicals, but if you overwhelm them with harmful chemicals (for example, from to-bacco smoke or from a city environment where the air usually contains high levels of car, airplane, and other exhausts containing benzene, a po-tent cancer-causing agent, as well as many other cancer-causing agents) they are far more likely to become diseased with primary lung cancer and far less likely to be able to fight against invading breast cancer cells trying to establish secondary tumors.

The liver is an amazing organ responsible for eliminating poisonous chemicals from the body, including those produced by our own meta-bolism, as well as manufacturing all sorts of important enzymes and other chemicals essential for our bodies to function. The liver detoxifies our system and produces anticancer chemicals. My strategy was, and continues to be, to eat as many good nutritious substances as possible to help my liver to help me, and to keep it as unburdened as possible with pollutants in my food, applied to my skin, or inhaled.

One of the main sources of pollutants to try to eliminate is tobacco smoke. It is estimated that smoking tobacco causes approximately 30 per-cent of all cancers in the United States alone. Smoking tobacco not only causes cancer in the lungs but is also implicated in cancer of the mouth, windpipe, esophagus, bladder, and pancreas and probably of the stomach, liver, and kidney. It may also contribute to some forms of leukemia, cancer of the colon, rectum, and other organs. Tobacco smoke is the single most lethal cancer-causing agent known. It contains more than 200 cancer-causing agents. These include radioactive substances such as po-lonium 210, highly poisonous heavy metals such as cadmium, and dangerous organic chemicals such as the polycyclic aromatic hydrocarbons (PAHs), which cause serious damage to DNA (see below). Heavy smoking on its own increases lung cancer risk by about 2,000 percent.[13] I have never smoked. I find that the cough most smokers develop, their brown teeth and thin wrinkly skin, not to mention their smell, is all I need to say no, and I try to avoid passive smoking. If people ask me if I mind if they smoke in my presence, I say yes. If you do smoke and are addicted to nicotine and find it difficult to give up, you can reduce your risks by having nicotine as patches or by chewing nicotine-impregnated gum—it is the tar in tobacco that contains the powerful cancer-causing agents, not the nicotine. I do not blame individual smokers for their habit. Such is the power of advertising and image that increasingly young people are persuaded to spend a lot of money taking up a habit that makes them become progressively less attractive for the rest of us to look at and smell, and potentially seriously ill.

I am now going to tell you about some other damaging chemicals in the environment before advising you on how to cut your exposure to them. The concentration of many of them, especially the endocrine-disrupting chemicals, can actually be measured by their effects on breast cancer cell cultures. Many are fat-soluble and bioaccumulate up the food chain, becoming especially concentrated in milk.

CANCER HAZARD: POLYCYCLIC AROMATIC HYDROCARBONS (PAHs)

These are formed by the incomplete combustion of other hydrocarbons. Because there are so many partial combustion processes that favor production of PAHs, they can be abundant in the atmosphere, soil, and elsewhere in the environment from sources that include engine exhausts, cigarette smoke, broiled food, and coal and wood smoke. Coal tars and petroleum residues such as road and roofing asphalt also have high levels of PAHs. Many contaminated land sites such as old gas works have high levels of PAHs.

They deserve special attention because some of them act as endocrine-disrupting chemicals (EDCs—see p. 222), and some cause cancer in other ways. What makes them particularly dangerous is their rather sinister chemical properties. In the environment they are very unreactive, which makes them persistent and difficult to get rid of. When they enter the human body, the liver tries to eliminate them, but oxidized PAH metabolites can react chemically and become permanently inserted into the structure of DNA, thereby introducing mistakes into it. It is the ability of PAH metabolites to become *intercalated* in, or slotted into, the DNA structure because of their limited chemical reactivity in the body that makes some PAH compounds so carcinogenic.

Their complicated name refers to the fact that they comprise more than one ring of carbon atoms. Benzene, which is the basic single-ring structure of carbon atoms with hydrogen atoms attached from which PAHs are built up, is itself a very powerful carcinogen. Some PAH compounds, including benzo[*a*]pyrene, whose molecules are arranged in five benzene rings and which is concentrated in tobacco smoke, are well known to be the precursors of cancer-causing metabolites.

Benzene has special regulations for its use in laboratories in order to meet Health and Safety regulations. So it always strikes me as strange that we are allowed to be exposed to this dangerous chemical every time we fill our cars with gas or walk down the street and breathe in car exhaust fumes or our own or other people's cigarette smoke.[14] Typical tests on exhaust fumes from cars show that they emit about 16 mg of benzene for every mile traveled.[15]

CANCER HAZARD: DIOXINS

The major source of dioxin in the environment (95 percent) is incinerators burning chlorinated wastes. Dioxin is formed as an unintentional by-product of many industrial processes involving chlorine, such as waste incineration, chemical and pesticide manufacturing, and pulp and paper bleaching. Dioxin pollution is also associated with the production of poly-vinyl chloride (PVC) plastics. Dioxin was the primary toxic component of Agent Orange, was found at Love Canal in Niagara Falls, New York, and was the basis for evacuation at Seveso, Italy, and the Bhopal disaster in India.

Dioxin (polychlorinated dibenzo-para-dioxins and dibenzofurans) is a general term that describes a group of hundreds of chemicals that are highly persistent in the environment. The most toxic compound is 2,3,7,8-tetra-chlorodibenzo-p-dioxin, or TCDD. The name dioxin is also used for the family of structurally and chemically related polychlorinated dibenzo-para-dioxins (PCDDs), polychlorinated dibenzofurans (PCDFs), and certain polychlorinated biphenyls (PCBs). Some 419 types of dioxin-related compounds have been identified, but only about 30 are considered to have significant toxicity, with TCDD being the most toxic.[16]

TCDD dioxin is, in fact, one of the most toxic chemicals known. According to a September 1994 report of the U.S. Environmental Protection Agency (EPA), not only does there appear to be no "safe" level of exposure to dioxin, but levels of dioxin and dioxin-like chemicals have been found in the general U.S. population that are "at or near levels associated with adverse health effects." The EPA report confirmed that dioxin is a cancer hazard to people; that exposure to dioxin can also cause severe reproductive and developmental problems (at levels 100 times lower than those associated with its cancer-causing effects); and that dioxin can cause immune system damage and interfere with regulatory hormones.

Short-term exposure of humans to high levels of dioxins may result in skin lesions, such as chloracne and patchy darkening of the skin, and altered liver function. Long-term exposure is linked to impairment of the immune system and reproductive functions. Chronic exposure of animals to dioxins has resulted in several types of cancer. The International Agency for Research on Cancer [IARC]—part of the World Health Organization—announced on 14 February 1997 that the most potent dioxin, 2,3,7,8-TCDD, is now considered a Class 1 carcinogen, meaning a "known human carcinogen."

According to the EPA's Health Assessment report, the Dioxin Reassessment Summary, dioxin is hydrophobic, fat-soluble, and bioaccumulates up the food chain; it is found mainly (97.5 percent) in meat and dairy products.[17] The North American intake based on a total exposure of 119 pg/day (a picogram [pg] is one trillionth of a gram) is as follows: dairy products and milk, 34 percent; beef, 32 percent; chicken, 11 percent; pork, 11 percent; fish, 7 percent; and eggs, 3 percent. Milk in the United Kingdom also contains dioxins and PCBs.[18]

Extensive stores of waste industrial oils with high levels of dioxins exist throughout the world. Long-term storage of this material may result in dioxin release into the environment and the contamination of human and animal food supplies. Dioxins are not easily disposed of without contamination of the environment and human populations.

Incineration is the best available method of destruction although other methods are being investigated. The process requires high temperatures (over 1562°F). For destruction of large amounts of contaminated material, even higher temperatures—1832°F or more—are required. Further information on dioxin is available on several websites including http://www.enviroweb.org/issues/dioxin/index.html and those of the World Wildlife Fund, the World Health Organization, and the EPA.

CANCER HAZARD: POLYCHLORINATED BIPHENYLS (PCBs)

The abbreviation PCB refers to a family of man-made chemicals that contains 209 individual compounds with varying toxicity. Commercial formulations of PCBs enter the environment as mixtures of a variety of PCBs and impurities. They have very high chemical, thermal, and biological stability, low vapor pressure, and are good electrical insulators and fire retardants. Between the 1930s and 1970s these properties led to the manufacture and use of PCBs as coolant-insulation fluids in transformers and capacitors, for the impregnation of cotton and asbestos, as plasticizers, and as additives to some epoxy paints. The same properties that made the extraordinarily stable PCBs so useful also contributed to their widespread dispersion and accumulation in the environment. The manufacture of PCBs was discontinued in the United States and their uses and disposal were strictly controlled after 1976.

It has been estimated that since 1929, a total of 1.2 million tons of PCBs have been manufactured.[19] Of this total, 31 percent (370,000 tons) have so far escaped into the general environment. An estimated 4 percent of original production have been fed into incinerators for intended destruction. However, 780,000 tons of PCBs are still in use in transformers and capacitors or have been sent to landfills. Thus the amount that could potentially be released into the environment is approximately twice as large as the amount that has already been released.

PCBs enter the body through contaminated food and air and through skin contact. They are found particularly in fatty food including milk.[20] Fish have been implicated, but a survey of fish products reported in 1997 indicated that fish liver oils contained higher concentrations of PCBs and dioxins than fish body oils, so fish are safer than fish oils.[21] Exposure from drinking water is minimal. It is known that nearly all humans have PCBs in their bodies, including infants who drink breast milk containing PCBs.[22] Animal experiments have shown that some PCB mixtures produce adverse health effects that include liver damage, skin irritations, reproductive and development effects, and cancer. Some PCBs cause mutations in cells, and they are endocrine disrupters (see p. 222). Therefore it is prudent to consider that there may be health hazards for humans.

While the risk of PCBs in producing cancer and reproductive and developmental effects in humans cannot be clearly defined, the suggestive evidence provides an additional basis for public health concern about humans who may be exposed to PCBs. The complexity of relating the specific mixtures for which data are available to exposures in the general population has resulted in a tendency to regard all PCBs as having a similar health hazard potential, although this assumption may not be true.

The U.S. Food and Drug Administration specifies limits on PCB concentration of 0.2 to 3 parts per million (milligrams of PCBs per kilogram of food) in infant foods, eggs, milk (in milk fat), and poultry (fat).

The EPA guideline for drinking water ranges from 0.005 to 0.5 mcg of PCBs per liter of water, which also reflects the risk of a person developing cancer of 1 in 10 million to 1 in 100,000.

In Britain, levels of PCBs in soils peaked in the late 1960s but have now fallen to the levels of the 1940s, and the estimated U.K. dietary intake of PCBs declined by about two thirds between 1982 and 1992.[23] Disposal of PCBs from discarded electrical equipment and other sources remains a problem.

CANCER HAZARD: ENDOCRINE-DISRUPTING CHEMICALS (EDCs)

One of the ways many pollutants are now implicated in causing cancer is in the way they have been shown to mimic hormones; hence they are called endocrine-disrupting chemicals (EDCs). (There is a move to call these chemicals endocrine modifiers, presumably because this plays down to the public the potential hazard that these chemicals represent.) Because breast and prostate cancer have been suggested to be hormonally controlled cancers, EDCs are of particular significance.

Residues from many pesticides, plastics, and household chemicals, such as detergents, that mimic hormones—including estrogens—leach into our food and water. They are fat-soluble and in the case of estrogenic EDCs have an estrogenic effect on the body because the body cannot distinguish the molecules from those of natural estrogen. In addition to estrogen-mimicking substances, other endocrine disrupters are thought to block estrogen, mimic or block androgens (male hormones), and possibly also mimic or block thyroid hormones. Because EDCs are related to hormones, an infinitesimal quantity can have a negative effect.[24] In the case of derivatives of persistent organochlorines and herbicides, which have a high residence period, they can accumulate in the body and be passed from one generation to the next.

The following substances, some of which we have discussed above, have been identified as environmental endocrine disrupters by the World Wildlife Fund and/or the EPA:

+ Persistent organochlorines (usually called polychlorinated dibenzo-*p*-dioxins/dibenzofurans [PCDD/PCDFs] or dioxins, furans, and PCBs)

+ Pesticides such as dichlorodiphenyltrichloroethane (DDT), lindane, malathion, atrazine, and simazine
+ Some polycyclic aromatic hydrocarbons (PAHs)
+ Lead and mercury
+ Some industrial chemicals such as butyl benzenes-P
+ Polymers such as polyurethane
+ Phthalates (used as plasticizers)
+ Alkyl phenols (surfactants or detergents)
+ Tributyl tin (antifouling agent used on ships and as a wood preservative)
+ Steroid hormones (from natural sources, the contraceptive pill, and hormone replacement therapy)

Although EDCs are of great interest to agencies responsible for determining their potential effects on humans and wildlife, it is expensive and difficult to monitor most of them in the environment. Some of the new methods designed to measure their concentrations and distribution in the environment and in biological samples actually use bioassay methods that depend upon the ability of the chemicals to stimulate cultures of breast cancer cells. For example, Shin and coworkers have used genetically modified human breast cancer (MCF-7) cells to show that nonylphenol—a breakdown product from detergents and plasticizers, bisphenol A—a plasticizer, pentachlorobiphenyl—a PCB, and DDT cause the breast cancer cell cultures to respond in a dose-dependent manner (i.e., the more EDC that is added to the breast cancer culture, the more the culture responds).[25] Also, A. M. Soto has shown that combinations of commonly encountered chemicals in the environment can have more than multiplicative effects on cultures of breast cancer cells.[26]

Xenoestrogens ("stranger" estrogens) in addition to altering estrogen metabolism can produce direct genetic damage throughout the cell cycle.[27] Some xenohormones or their metabolites can produce free radicals or otherwise indirectly modify DNA structure or function.

Some researchers have suggested that xenoestrogens are unlikely to cause harm because we are already exposed to phytoestrogen chemicals. Humans are likely to have evolved defenses against harm from phytoestrogens, however. Moreover, bioaccumulative persistent xenoestrogens and other endocrine disrupters accumulate in body tissues to much higher levels than phytoestrogens.[28] All the epidemiological and other research I have read suggests that phytoestrogens are protective against breast cancer while xenoestrogens are potentially harmful.

The situation has not been helped by the fact that many doctors take little or no interest in the environment and often do not know much about the chemicals used in industry, agriculture, or even in the home environment, or their effects. For example, an article in the October 1999 issue of the *British Medical Journal* implied that crop yields would go on increasing, but there was no mention of the input of chemicals that this would require.[29] The article stated:

> Since 1945 the United States and Canada (with Australia) have been the world's most important exporters of cereals. The average growth of yields in these countries has been and remains strong. For example in the United States the average cereal yield rose from 4.58 tonnes per hectare in 1989–91 to 5.04 tonnes per hectare in 1995–7. There is no reason to believe that average yields will not continue to rise at a reasonable absolute rate.

There is no mention in the article of the pesticides and other chemicals that have been used to achieve the increase in yield. I have served on committees and attended many meetings concerned with the environment and health. At one meeting I recall that all the environmentalists sat through the presentations given by the medical specialists, but the doctors all left before any of the papers on the environment were presented. Thank goodness for doctors such as Professor A. J. McMichael at the London School of Health and Tropical Hygiene, author of the book *Planetary Overload* (CUP, 1993), who has developed a broader vision of the causes of ill health related to the environment—including the industrialization of agriculture—and pollution.

According to a European Environment Agency (EEA)/United Nations Environment Program (UNEP) report published in 1999 entitled "Chemicals in the European Environment: Low Doses, High Stakes," there are now many thousands of (man-made) chemicals on the market, and little is known about their fate or impact on people or the environment. The EEA/UNEP report states that such chemicals are widespread in the air, soil, water, and stream, river, and coastal sediments of Europe following the marketing, use, disposal, and degradation of about 100,000 novel substances since the 1950s. Monitoring of a few of these substances is required by law in the United States and Europe. However, since much of the monitoring involves analysis of water samples and since many of the compounds of concern are fat-soluble, not water-soluble, the monitoring schemes are likely to underestimate their true impact and presence in the environment. This means that, for many of these chemicals, we have no systematic data on their concentration or distribution in the environment. We also know next to nothing about methods of exposure, about their effect on the environment, and about their effect on human health. And we know nothing about the chemicals as they break down in the environment or in the body (metabolites).

In some cases, for example that of pesticides, release to the environment has been deliberate (although the consequences were often not foreseen and not recognized for many years). In other cases releases have been an unfortunate side effect of the use of substances by the manufacturing industry. In addition, harmful organic chemicals have accumulated in the environment because of energy generation, especially the combustion of fossil fuels. In some cases chemical releases have caused major incidents— for example, the release of dioxins at Love Canal in Niagara Falls, New York, and Seveso, Italy—but contamination is usually a more insidious process.

Let me quickly summarize how I and many other earth and environmental scientists see the situation.

Life on Earth has evolved in a complex interrelationship with the environment for at least 3,500 million years. Modern man, whose body chemistry has developed over that period of biological evolution, has appeared in the last ten-thousandth of the planet's history (equivalent to the last ten seconds on the 24-hour clock). In the past fifty years or so (much less than a fraction of a second on the 24-hour clock) we have set about dramatically changing the types and proportions of chemical molecules in the environment.

In particular, we have reconfigured organic chemicals, which were the basis of all life, into new "organic" substances to use in industry and industrialized agriculture. In some cases the new "organic" substances (which range from plastics to pesticides), their by-products, or their metabolites are the *antithesis* of life. Some of the new chemicals and their by-products are implicated in causing cancer. Chemicals that disrupt the endocrine system by which chemical messengers or hormones control our physiological function are of particular concern in breast and prostate cancer.

MAKING SENSE OF IT ALL—THE PRACTICALITIES

I try to have as few man-made chemicals in my life as possible. I cannot live without my makeup, but I use hypoallergenic products. In the United States in 1990 (the latest figures available) 38,000 patients had cosmetic-related health problems, including contact dermatitis, asthma, and nausea requiring medical attention. One of the most extreme cases involved a woman whose bone marrow was affected by chemicals in hair dye to the extent that the level of her blood platelets dropped (not very helpful, especially if you are on chemotherapy).

I do not wear perfume and I use unperfumed simple soap and un-perfumed deodorant. I recently read the label on some expensive shower gel marketed by a prestigious company, to find that it actually listed phthalates—one of the main groups of endocrine disrupters implicated in the feminization of fish—among the chemicals it contained. Research by Professor John Sumpter of Brunel University, London, now suggests that parabens (a very common preservative in cosmetics) could be an estrogen-mimic (EDC—see p. 222).[30] With cosmetics, as with all other products: read the label, and remember, simpler is better.

I do not add chemicals other than simple salts such as Epsom salts to my bathwater. Even familiar man-made chemicals are often eventually shown to cause problems. A recent report in the magazine *Nature* suggests that a commonly used antibacterial agent, triclosan, may work by causing mutations in bacteria.[31] Triclosan is used in many antibacterial soaps, lotions, mouthwash, toothpaste, plastic toys, socks, and cutting boards. I prefer to use good old-fashioned soap, not complex detergents or per-fumed soaps, which will bind with dirt, fat-soluble chemicals, and "germs" and wash them away.

I do not use chemicals to stay young artificially. I do not and would not take hormone replacement therapy, especially based on unopposed estrogen. Some doctors in America and at some London clinics are reportedly providing their patients with human growth hormone (the human equivalent of BST or BGH-1) to prevent aging. A study published in the *British Medical Journal* in 1998 reported that high natural levels of the hormone could lead to premature death from cancer. Also, growth hormones available to athletes and body builders must be of concern.

Many other cancer-causing agents have been identified, mainly as a result of occupational exposure—for example, of factory workers, painters and decorators, and hairdressers—to high levels of particular chemical substances. Some of the most dangerous chemicals implicated include benzene (used in the manufacture of some furniture and rubber and emitted from some types of fresh paint and car exhausts), formaldehyde (often used as a preservative; for example, on fabrics in new cars, clothes, and furnishings and in some cosmetics and shampoos), hair dyes, and PCBs in transformers, hydraulic fluids, some paints and varnishes, lubricants, some inks, adhesives, and insecticides.[32]

I have my hair streaked, but this does not involve having chemicals applied directly onto the scalp. I would avoid using hair dyes, especially certain dark-colored ones; some of these contain chemicals suspected of causing cancer when applied directly to the scalp. Discuss this with your hairdressers and ensure that they have checked the information on the carcinogenicity of any chemicals they use.

One of the alternative therapies I question as a treatment for cancer is aromatherapy, especially if you are undergoing chemotherapy. Your liver already has a massive job to do to clear out all the unwanted chemicals, dead cells, and other debris from the treatment without having to deal with other powerful chemicals. The skin is the body's largest organ, and a proportion of many of the things we put on it is absorbed into the bloodstream.

In aromatherapy a carrier oil such as almond oil (thought not to be absorbed by the skin) is used as a base, and an essential oil that normally evaporates (and has molecules that can pass through the skin) is added to achieve particular effects. Some of the oils absorbed through the skin (transdermally) are concentrated extracts of powerful chemicals. Many people wrongly believe that because the essential oils used in aromatherapy are extracted from plants and flowers they cannot be harmful, despite being delivered in high concentrations through the skin. In nature they are at low concentrations as part of a total fruit, flower, or leaf. Many of the essential oils have never been tested scientifically for their side effects, but medical research has shown that camphor, hyssop, and sage oils can have such serious side effects as causing fits. Limonene—the lemon-smelling aromatherapy oil—is known to be capable of causing kidney damage. Basil oil, which is said to lift mood, and tarragon oil also contain a chemical called estrogole, which causes cancer in rodents. Dr. Sharon Hopkiss of the Department of Pharmacology and Toxicology at Saint Mary's Hospital Medical School in London has been quoted as saying that many oils used in aromatherapy are extremely potent natural agents.

The only car I drive is an old Land Rover of 1972 vintage with an engine converted to use lead-free gasoline. If anything goes wrong we simply buy a new part and put it in. Any volatile organic chemicals used in its manufacture or sprayed on its interior will long since have evaporated. Even so, I try to use it as little as possible and usually travel by public transport. The chemicals emitted by cars, even when well tuned and running optimally, include many hazardous substances such as benzene (see John Pearson's book *The Air Quality Challenge*). If you paint your house or have it painted, ensure that it is well ventilated (some of the oil-based paints used in Britain are now banned in Scandinavia). Also, new furniture, curtains, and upholstery can be important sources of formaldehyde and benzene, and benzene is given off by many fast-drying glues. Polyvinyl chlorides (PVCs) should also be avoided as much as possible. In an article in *The* (London) *Times* of 11 November 1999 by Martin Fletcher, it was reported that the European Commission had called for an emergency ban on soft PVC toys, including rattles and pacifiers, which babies suck. It was claimed that these contained dangerous chemicals. Again the dangerous chemicals concerned were phthalates. The report claimed that eight EU states had already banned phthalates from toys, but Britain was not among them. It went on to point out that phthalates are used for softening the plastic.

If some plant in my garden is going to die, so be it. I will feed it with composted household waste to help it survive, but I minimize my use of chemicals around the house or in the garden. My garden has lots of different wild bird species, butterflies, ladybugs, toads, and hedgehogs. The degree of biodiversity in my garden compared with those of many friends who use chemicals says a great deal about the damage our use of chemicals does to the animals, so why do we think that we will be un-affected? We have already discussed problems associated with pesticides implicated in breast cancer. Although I know of no evidence that organ-ophosphates are carcinogenic, they are damaging to the central nervous system. In addition to sheep dip and shampoos to kill head lice, many familiar products are based on organophosphates. They include many in-secticides, sprays, and treatments for lice or fleas on pets, including flea collars. I avoid all these products. I never use aerosol sprays for hair, deodorants, cleaning, gardening, or any other purpose because of the in-creased risk of inhaling man-made chemicals.

I use wood, glass, ceramics, and natural mineral materials in my home; stainless steel, enamel, or toughened glass for cooking; and alu-minium foil to wrap food. I use natural materials for clothing and furnishing whenever I can, with as few plastics, man-made fibers, or other chemicals in my life as possible. Also, I always wash and thoroughly rinse new clothes before wearing them to remove preservatives. I also minimize my use of detergents and ensure that they are thoroughly rinsed from dishes and clothes before use. You might find it strange that someone who has spent her professional career working in chemical laboratories should try so hard to avoid them in everyday life. Like many of my colleagues, I have a healthy respect for what chemicals can do to biological processes and so minimize my exposure.

If you eat good nutritious food and reduce exposure to pollutants, you will find that your skin and general appearance improve without the need to add polluting man-made chemicals to your body or the environ-ment. We can all reduce our personal risk from hazardous chemicals, and by doing so we help the environment generally, with cleaner water and soils and hence more wholesome food. To most natural scientists this is all just common sense and is very easy to live with.

It is impossible to entirely eliminate risk from man-made chemical substances, but you can reduce your personal risk by following the guide-lines above, and whenever you read or hear a new advertisement for a new beauty product, man-made fabric, or garden spray, for example, think very carefully about whether you really need it. Almost certainly you do not. People who avoid such products are frequently portrayed as odd, especially by those wishing to make money by selling us products that we do not need. No one looking at me, spending time with me, or visiting my home would think I was a crank. Unless it was pointed out to them, they probably would not notice anything missing or different. Indeed, most people comment on how normal I am—presumably despite being a scientist!

All the factors described in Chapters 5 and 6 are easy to control in your own surroundings. I also travel a lot internationally, and here are a few tips to help you maintain The Plant Program while on your travels.

AWAY FROM HOME

1. When traveling, allow plenty of time for every aspect of the journey. Do not allow yourself to become stressed or upset by delays. If flying, try to fly at night to cut your exposure to cosmic radiation.
2. Count out the number of kelp, brewer's yeast, and red clover tablets to cover you for your entire time away and take a small pot of dried soy milk (normally sold in cans for babies and infants). Take herbal tea bags and enough fruit to see you through until you can find a local supply.
3. When flying, ensure that you order a vegan meal and check that the travel agent uses the code VGML, as other codes can include dairy. Drink lots of boiled water flavored with your own herbal tea bags to avoid dehydration. Drink beer to make you sleepy.
4. Travel only on No Smoking flights or in No Smoking train compartments.
5. When you arrive at your destination, locate the nearest fruit and vegetable shop and buy fresh supplies daily. In many countries these must be washed in boiling water before eating. This is really a brief immersion (use the hotel sink) similar to the blanching process used in cooking. (Many hotels provide kettles or boiling water on request.)
6. Before you travel, look up key words in a dictionary and jot them down in the language of the country you will be visiting. For example, in France soy is *soja*. Having a small number of

ready-translated words at hand will greatly ease your visit. Ask your hotel where to buy the items you need, using the written version if necessary. There will usually be a supermarket near your hotel where you can buy supplies, including beer, and thus avoid using the hotel's expensive minibar.

7. Research the local cuisine and check which dishes you will be able to eat without problem or fuss.

8. Tell everyone you are terribly allergic to dairy products and insist that you have none at all. (I have found this is most difficult in France.) If all else fails you can remove the cheese or scrape off the yogurt or cream—I do so ostentatiously!

9. Be inventive in avoiding dairy products. For example, at the breakfast buffet use prune or other fruit juice to moisten your cereal.

10. If you have trouble sleeping in a different time zone, chamomile is soothing and beer always makes me sleepy.

7.

Reflections from
West to East

---

*In this chapter I explain why "the system" has failed to protect us
from, or even inform us of, many avoidable risk factors implicated
in breast and prostate cancer. It explains why I have come to the
conclusion that women must to a great extent rely on themselves in
matters of health. Your life really is in your hands. You become
empowered by knowledge. The facts and scientific insights provided
in this book are intended to reduce risk—for the individual and
for society. In conclusion, I suggest Ten Golden Guidelines for you
to follow.*

I believe that in this book I have put together compelling evidence of the
likely causes of breast and prostate cancer and then developed methods
for modifying diet and lifestyle that have the potential to greatly reduce
the threat that these diseases represent.

But one thing still greatly puzzles and disturbs me.

All the information, scientific experiments, epidemiology, surveys,
and research you've just read have been published in respected, peer-
reviewed scientific journals. In many cases this information has been available for years, even decades.

Q Why haven't we been told about it?

A As a scientist, I read quite widely: numerous general scientific journals, as well as specialist journals in my own field. And I read the usual newspapers, watch television programs, and generally keep as up-to-date as most people do. And yet, before contracting breast cancer, I'd never heard of any of this vital information.

Q Why not?

A True, the media are full of information and advice on breast cancer, but most of it is either simplistic, unscientific, or conflicting. I have *never* seen anything about the case against dairy products that is set out here, or much about the connection with endocrine-disrupting chemicals. Who else has made these connections—and why has no one in authority acted on them?

Let us consider what has happened in other situations that involve commercial products that affect our health.

Many elements of the Western diet are known to cause ill health; for example, the high levels of cholesterol and triglycerides in butter, cheese, and meat have been linked to heart disease for a very long time. Yet the public has never been given a clear explanation of the risks. In presenting the results of the China study we examined earlier in Chapter 3, Campbell and Junshi showed that even small intakes of food of animal origin are associated with significant increases in plasma cholesterol concentrations, which are associated, in turn, with significant increases in chronic degenerative diseases (cardiovascular, diabetes, and several types of cancer including breast and colon cancer).[1] They noted that in the West, reduction in fat consumption was being achieved by using lower-fat foods (e.g., low-fat dairy foods, leaner cuts of meat, less added fat), while the fruit-vegetable-cereal recommendation appeared to have received little attention—even though these foods contain virtually *all* the individual constituents known to prevent chronic degenerative disease. Concerned by this highly selective distortion of their important message, the scientists speculate that pressure from food industry lobbying groups has influenced both the media (and hence public perception) and also those who set official policy. I have to say that this seems to be the most likely explanation. The situation is of particular concern since, as we discussed on

p. 126, animal proteins as well as fats are now being implicated in cancer and heart disease.

Instead of developing good risk-communication methods aimed at disease prevention, we continue to treat disease with pills and potions, surgery, or other expensive, invasive methods to suppress symptoms. Communicating problems in our diet and lifestyle that affect our health is typically done poorly—or not at all—and usually without clear advice on how to change our behavior.

This whole approach avoids antagonizing special interest groups, and it maintains the material wealth of (and jobs in) sectors such as farming, agrochemicals, the food industry, pharmaceutical research, and the manufacture of medicines and medical equipment. But would it not be better to communicate facts as they are known, clearly and simply, so that people can make their own choices and prevent disease? Would it not be better to create jobs in sectors working for the well-being of society and the environment—for example, in growing wholesome, nutritious, organically produced food, with medical professionals being concerned more with health education, disease prevention, and monitoring than dishing out pills? The effectiveness of this approach has been demonstrated dramatically by the decrease in the numbers of people in the United Kingdom dying of lung cancer because they have quit smoking.[2]

WHERE DOES THE FAULT LIE?

I believe that much of the problem lies in the genuine lack of understanding of science among politicians. Very few politicians are scientists. Most of them have degrees in law, politics, or economics, and many frequently appear more concerned that their country retain its competitive edge economically than with public health or the environment. Wealth creation generally takes precedence over quality of life, which I suspect reflects the views of most of their constituents.

In the United States, according to Derek Bok, until recently President of Harvard University, "Universities are constantly pressed to accept questionable arrangements with industry [which may include] provisions prohibiting academic scientists funded by one company from collaborating with investigators funded by another. A few institutions have even agreed to clauses that require them to keep faculty members from speaking about their commercially funded research at academic meetings without first submitting their remarks to their industry sponsors."[3]

Many industries have sponsored university research as part of a policy of blunting the impact of adverse findings associated with their products. The most fully documented example is that of the tobacco companies misleading the public over the risks associated with smoking. The tobacco industry kept secret its own findings, dating from the early 1960s, that nicotine was addictive and that smoking probably caused cancer. To protect its commercial interests it funded special "public science" contracts with universities in Britain as well as the United States. These were designed to carry out research in areas where evidence might be found that showed tobacco in a better light and that could then be used to create controversy over the "alleged" dangers of smoking. The source of funding for this research was not publicly disclosed. When eventually in 1994 the details of this campaign became known, the tobacco industry used all the weapons available to a powerful industry to try to suppress their publication. This included attempting to stop a university library from holding the documents in stock, seeking to obtain from the library a list of all the readers who had consulted the documents, and using party political influence in an endeavor to cut off the research funds of the academic involved.[4]

The problem of conflict of interest in relation to the food industry is discussed at length by Dr. R. M. Kradjian,[5] who gives examples of what he suggest are dubious research findings linked to funding from the dairy industry. In the last chapter of his book he concludes:

> Much of our highly varied, desired, and profitable food supply has been found to be dangerous. The people who furnish this food and who are enriched by its sale do not want you to know this. They have generously contributed to scientists who have supported, and are willing to continue to support, their products. If those scientists suddenly have a change of heart, and seriously challenge the safety of that food, you may be certain that the bulk of the food-industry financial support will promptly disappear.
>
> Whom are you going to believe? Those with no financial gain from the sale of food and with the backing of the world's scientific

literature? Or are you going to follow those who have at times devised flawed studies and reaped millions of dollars in support from the industries that they fail to seriously criticize? You must decide, and your health will be substantially determined by your decision.

Even government-funded research—which should be conspicuously in the public interest and, surely, freely available to every citizen—all too often seems to be regarded as a tool of policy. If the research supports the existing or proposed policy, fine. But if not, then it may typically be subject to any or all of the following:[6]

+ No press release or press conference
+ Not published through usual departmental channels
+ Only duplicated copies of typescript available in minimal numbers
+ Timed to be released on the Friday before a weekend or holiday.

The bovine spongiform encephalopathy (BSE) or "mad cow" crisis was a prime example of the way in which public-interest science can be concealed, distorted, or misrepresented. Problems included secrecy of "scientific" meetings, partial publication of research results, the implied threat to future research funding, and the vilification of critics or, indeed, any concerned scientist.[7] According to Sheila Jasanoff, Professor of Science and Technology Studies at Cornell University, "What made the news so appalling was not just the thought that beef, a staple of British diets, could be fatally contaminated. It was not even that CJD [Creutzfeldt-Jakob disease] struck without notice, was incurable, and caused a horrifying death. It was that, since 1988, the government and some of its advisers had repeatedly stated that beef was safe, a formulation widely taken to mean that transmission of BSE from cows to people was impossible. If government officials had deliberately misled the public, then how could anything they now said be trusted?"[8]

Scientists are increasingly concerned about the poor image they have in Britain following fiascos such as the BSE crisis, for which they are unfairly blamed by politicians and public alike. But their image will only improve when we adopt official policies that have far greater transparency, and when public scientists regain the public's respect for forthright and straightforward impartiality.

Clinical doctors, too, must develop far more awareness and interest in diet, lifestyle, and the environment. The fact that many of the doctors I know do not eat healthy diets suggests that they do not know the importance of good nutrition. Let me describe what happened to John Camac. John was so impressed by my recovery that he put many of his patients suffering from breast cancer, including a close friend of one of his daughters, in touch with me and strongly suggested that they follow my advice. However, he could not bring himself to do this himself. He lived on a traditional Western diet with very few vegetables. He refused to eat any cruciferous vegetables; the only green vegetables I ever persuaded him to eat were peas. He suffered progressively from a series of degenerative diseases—diabetes, arthritis, coronary heart disease, which was treated with a heart bypass—and he finally died of liver cancer. To deal with his symptoms he took an increasing range and quantity of pills prescribed by what he described as "top specialists in their field." The only food or drink he used to help his health was red wine for his heart, which Western medicine seems to believe in. By the time he was prepared to listen to me it was far too late, although shortly before he died he was drinking juices and eating soy. I still recollect visiting him in the hospital after his heart bypass operation when he was offered a choice of several drinks by a nurse. I urged him to choose orange juice, but he drank a large glass of milk. He died of liver cancer six months after his heart bypass operation.

Very few of my friends who are medical professionals seem to know much about food chemistry, and I have often seen consultants and junior doctors at Charing Cross Hospital buying junk food. It is my impression that they are all so busy that they do not have time to eat a proper lunch, probably because they work such long hours under intense pressure. All my observations tell me that most doctors are unaware of the likely connections between the food we consume, chemicals in our environment, and breast and prostate cancer. Instead, much of their knowledge is based on the literature they are bombarded with about new drugs and procedures. I think it is unrealistic to expect clinical doctors—who are incredibly busy trying to meet targets imposed on them by politicians to assuage public concern—to root out all the scientific literature on breast cancer that I have found. Anyway, even if I am right and we now know the cause of breast cancer, will we change our behavior or will we still expect to consume what we want and then expect doctors to pick up the pieces? Experience of what we have done with our knowledge of the dangers of smoking, which we have had for at least forty years, suggests that the latter is more likely. Some people still continue to smoke regularly throughout their lives, despite knowing the risks, and then expect doctors to treat them for the range of cancers, including lung cancer, and other diseases caused by smoking tobacco.

My answer to the question "Whose fault is the breast and prostate cancer epidemic?" is that it is the fault of all of us—especially the relatively well-educated women and men in society. It is also my view that we are the ones who must make the changes that will reduce both our personal and societal risk of suffering from these diseases.

OUR LIVES IN OUR HANDS

It was thanks to a particularly unusual set of circumstances that I was able to join up many of the pieces of research into the causes of breast and prostate cancer and develop methods of preventing and treating the disease. These included my experience of working in China and Korea and to a lesser extent with Japanese, Taiwanese, and Thai colleagues and my good fortune in being given *The Atlas of Cancer Mortality in the People's Republic of China* and having many opportunities to talk to Chinese and other Eastern scientific colleagues. I am grateful to have had the scientific training to fight my way through the scientific jargon and to have found the strength to withstand the disease, develop methods of treating it, and finally cure myself. Even the controversy about the use of bovine soma-totropin in milk production helped my understanding of problem chemicals in milk.

Timing was also important. I was lucky enough to travel to Hong Kong, Beijing, and Seoul when Western influence on the local diets was less marked. Had I been only recently, I would not have realized the traditional differences between Eastern and Western diets. I always used to enjoy eating in China, Japan, or Korea because I could relax knowing that the food was safe for me. Lately I have become very concerned when I have revisited China and Korea to see the amount of Western junk food that is now consumed there, especially by young people. They have been persuaded by advertising and marketing that it is sophisticated to drink strongly promoted Western fizzy drinks and to eat burgers made from processed dairy cows, butter, and salads covered with the pale yellow or pale pink glop that is usually dumped over salads and sandwiches in North America unless you insist beforehand that you do not want it. Increasingly, Eastern people now eat chocolate puddings covered in cream and end their meals with chocolate and coffee with cream, although they still do not appear to eat much cheese. Food shopping and eating in Beijing used to be a great pleasure for me, but when I last visited my favorite supermarket, it was full of typical Western processed junk food and I had to search very hard to find even soy milk! In Hong Kong last year it was difficult to find truly traditional Chinese food in the area around my hotel. No wonder rates of breast and prostate cancer are rising in Eastern countries.

In this book I have given information to reduce the individual's risk of breast and prostate cancer, but the only lasting answer to these scourges of our Western lifestyle is to *change* that lifestyle. We have to develop greater awareness of, and sensitivity to, the impact of our lifestyle choices on our own health, that of our fellow beings, and that of our planetary home. Let me quote from Professor McMichael of the London School of Tropical Hygiene and Health and Dr. Powles of Cambridge University; their paper in a recent volume of the *British Medical Journal* states:[9]

Population size and the material intensity of our economies are now so great that, at the global level, we are disrupting some of the biosphere's life support systems. These systems provide the natural processes of stabilisation, replenishment, organic production, cleansing, and recycling that our predecessors were able to take for granted in a less populated, less disrupted world. We no longer live in such a world. We are changing the gaseous composition of the atmosphere: there is a net loss of productive soils on all continents: we have overfished most ocean fisheries: we have severely depleted many great aquifers on which irrigated agriculture depends; and we are extinguishing at an unprecedented overall rate whole species and many local populations. These changes to Earth's basic life supporting processes pose long term, and somewhat unfamiliar, risks to human health. Meanwhile the accompanying increases in local environmental pollutant levels, especially urban air pollution, exacerbate more familiar risks to health.

The authors could also have mentioned the industrialization of agriculture requiring the use of many chemicals to produce ever-increasing crop, milk, and meat yields and the future risks posed by genetically modified organisms if full risk analysis is not carried out for each product and their combinations. They conclude:

> Overall the larger potential threat is not from the increase in human numbers in itself but from today's globally averaged, mildly environmentally disruptive humans becoming highly disruptive—that is, from attempts to generalise production and consumption patterns typical of today's rich countries. Recent attempts at 'full cost accounting' estimate that the demands of the current world population already exceed global carrying capacity by approximately a third.
>
> The 'living planet' index is one of the first systematic attempts to quantify the effects of human activity on natural ecosystems. It gives equal weight to three contributing indices: forest ecosystems (area of natural forest cover) and freshwater ecosystems and marine ecosystems (trends in the population of 70 and 87 indicator species, respectively). Set to 100 in 1970, it was estimated to have fallen to 68 by 1995—an unsustainable rate of decline.
>
> Accordingly, a shift of emphasis from income to other types of wealth, especially stocks of human resources, improves the scope for enhancing health at any given level of income which is particularly important if we are to maximise human well-being while minimising consumption which leads to degradation and pollution of the planet.

What they are saying is that, if we are to survive as a healthy species, we must change our values and emphasis from materialism to other measures of well-being. We need increasingly to put more value on good food, education, the arts, beautiful unspoilt environments populated by diverse species other than man, friendships, social interaction, and health than on "things."

Looking back, I realize that I have changed from an ambitious middle-class, career-minded Western woman to a woman with a more traditional Eastern diet, lifestyle, and values. Here are some simple, practical guidelines that we can all follow to help us as individuals and as a society to cut our risk of breast and prostate cancer and probably many other noncommunicable or degenerative diseases, and improve our health at the same time.

MY TEN GOLDEN GUIDELINES

1. Make good food ingredients your top priority when it comes to spending money. Keep as closely as you can to The Plant Program and wherever and whenever possible be prepared to pay extra for organically grown food produced as naturally as possible or grow your own. This sends the clearest possible message to government and the food industry.

2. Eat only those foods that human adults have evolved to eat. Most crucially leave out dairy products, which are designed for baby calves, goats, or lambs. Also, refuse to eat food depleted of nutrients or otherwise altered by food processing, including food that contains artificial chemical additives such as coloring and flavoring agents, preservatives, and emulsifiers or food that has been chemically altered, such as fats that have been hydrogenated. Refuse to be bamboozled by marketing and advertising. Look for the "weasel words" and separate them in your mind from the underlying facts. Be suspicious—check labels and demand information.

3. Make eating good nutritious meals based on wholesome nutritional ingredients your top priority when it comes to your time. Saving money to acquire material possessions to demonstrate a sophisticated lifestyle and saving time to further your career ambitions are probably two of the fundamental causes of breast cancer in career women. One of my favorite novels is George Eliot's *Middlemarch*, and I continually strive to become more like Dorothea and less like Rosamund!

4. Be concerned and take action to improve the environment for everybody. There are many chemicals being introduced that we can do nothing about as individuals. Collectively, we *can* reduce the impact of chemicals on the environment by reducing our use

of materials such as perfumes and cosmetics, soft plastics, detergents, cleaning products and house and garden chemicals, and man-made fibers. Remember how in the past we were sold "wonder" chemicals such as DDT and PCBs, which have turned out to cause serious problems to the health of man, animals, and the environment and which are still with us. What chemicals are we using today that scientists will have a similar view of in the future? Press for more research into links between the evironment, nutrition, and human health and increased emphasis on epidemiological studies and disease prevention.

5. Try to understand some basic science. Usually it is *your* money that scientists are spending directly or indirectly and you need to understand what they are doing. Ensure that scientists contribute more to the public understanding of science by asking questions. If you do not understand the answer, do not be embarrassed to repeat your question until you get a satisfactory answer. If scientists cannot explain their work properly, it is their problem, not yours. Women in particular frequently throw up their hands at the very mention of science and say how unscientific they are—as if to admit knowing anything about science is unfeminine. It is essential that a well-informed body of opinion exist if science is to be directed toward the benefit of humankind rather than lead to our downfall. It is vital that women in particular be involved in the direction of science for the good of society. Books that will fire you up are *Silent Spring* by Rachel Carson; *Our Stolen Futures* by Colborn, Dumanski, and Myers; and *Planetary Overload* by A. J. McMichael. If you want to become more involved as lay members of the boards of scientific organizations, write in and offer your services.

6. Learn to understand your basic anatomy and carry out self-examination of your breasts at least once a month. Use books about the human body (there are some good, clear books aimed at children) to learn about your body, and ask the doctor or nurse at your local health center to show you how to examine yourself thoroughly. Do your examination a few days after your period ends, to ensure you know how your body looks and feels when it is normal, so that you will learn how not to bother your

doctor with nonproblems but get attention as soon as possible if there is a problem. This is particularly important if you are over 40. Also, if you are over 40 try to arrange a check of your breasts by a doctor or nurse once a year.

7. If the worst happens and you are diagnosed with breast cancer, use all the tools at your disposal to fight back. For your orthodox treatment, be sure you are treated at a center of excellence that uses a specialist cancer team led by a surgeon, radiation therapist, and chemotherapist. Work with your doctors and be an involved and constructive participant in overcoming your illness, not a passive victim.

8. Follow my diet and the lifestyle recommendations aimed at avoiding man-made chemicals as closely as possible. This includes minimizing the use of prescriptions available from doctors and pills from pharmacists. If drugs are prescribed or recommended, demand to know precisely how they work and what the side effects are. Take them only if you are satisfied with the explanation and convinced there is no alternative. If your physician cannot explain how the drugs work and give examples of their successes and failures, be skeptical.

9. Use methods such as meditation, hypnotherapy, visualization, and yoga to cope with emotional distress and develop the most positive approach possible. But do not rely on positive thinking alone. It is changing your body chemistry by changing your diet and lifestyle that is the crucial thing to do. Talk to your friends and family members and allow their help and support into your life, but if they find difficulty in coping, understand that they are distressed. Forgive them and allow them back into your life as soon as they feel able to return.

10. Breast cancer is *not* an automatic death sentence. Keep reminding yourself that *it is* possible to overcome even advanced cancer. Believe me. I did it.

Knowledge is power. In this book I have tried to empower *all* women to deal with breast cancer, individually and as a society, by trying to share with them the knowledge that I have gained on the subject of breast cancer as a scientist and as a five-times breast cancer sufferer.

Before my first diagnosis of cancer I was a go-getting career woman, and although I always made time for my children, I was a woman who had not only young children but a full-time job. I had become ill nourished because of reading food-industry (so called health) propaganda. I had survived on what was marketed and advertised as health food, albeit low fat and high fiber with large quantities of dairy food: cottage cheese and yogurt and dishes made using ground meat from slaughtered dairy cows, washed down with milky tea or commercial orange juice. I ate lots of fruit and cereals but few salads or vegetables. I simply took high-dose vitamin C pills and multivitamin, multimineral pills to cover any deficiencies.

I am now kinder to myself and to other people. I ensure that however hurried I am, however simple my meals, they are based on sound nutritional values. I now make time for family and friends and—amazingly—I seem to be even more successful in my work and my life. I am no longer a "fashion victim" in my clothes, home, garden, or car and I try to be as unmaterialistic as possible.

Instead, I am increasingly concerned with the environment and the sustainability of the surface of the beautiful blue planet called Earth as a place to live. Breast cancer changed me: from being insecure and easily persuaded by authority into a stronger woman who is her own person.

It made me stop.

And smell the (wild) roses. . . .

Notes

WELCOME

1. Selected causes of death: by gender and age. Office for National Statistics; General Register Office for Scotland; Northern Ireland Statistics and Research Agency, 1997.
2. Deaths: selected causes (International Classification) and sex, 1971 onwards (England and Wales): *Health Statistics Quarterly* 04, 1998.
3. http://who-pcc.iarc.fr/
4. Trichopoulos, Dimitrios; Li, Frederick P.; and Hunter, David J., 1996. What causes cancer? *Scientific American*, Special Issue, What You Need to Know about Cancer, September, 80–5.

CHAPTER 1

1. Plant, Jane A., and Moore, P.J., 1979. Geochemical mapping and interpretation in Britain. *Philosophical Transactions of the Royal Society, London,* B288, 95–112.
2. Plant, Jane A., and others, 2000. *Environmental Geochemistry at the Global Scale.* Geological Society Special Issue.
3. Dewey, John F., 1999. Society awards, *Geoscientist* 9, 6 June, 2–4.
4. Rennie, J., and Rusting, R., 1996. Making headway against cancer. *Scientific*

American, Special Issue, What You Need to Know about Cancer, September, 56–9.

5. Peto, R., and others, 2000. Smoking, smoking cessation, and lung cancer in the UK since 1950: combination of national statistics with two case-control studies. *British Medical Journal* 321, 323–9.

6. Raleigh, V.S., 1999. World population and health in transition. *British Medical Journal* 319, 981–4.

7. Packham, D.E., 1999. Impacts of commercialisation and privatisation on capabilities for scientific advice: oracles or scapegoats? IPMS Conference notes, October. See also Packham, David, and Tasker, Mary, 1997. Industry and the academy—a Faustian contract. *Industry and Higher Education*, April, 85–90.

8. See the World Health Organization's International Agency for Research on Cancer website: http://who-pcc.iarc.fr/

9. Physicians Committee for Responsible Medicine: PCRM Update of Winter 1991.

10. Cancer Research Campaign Factsheet 6.2, 1996.

11. Depression is very common—over two million people a year report symptoms. If you are a sufferer, first try to identify whether it is caused by real problems. If it is, get practical help in sorting them out—the Citizen's Advice Bureau is an excellent source of free advice on financial and legal problems, and Samaritans or friends can often help you to address emotionally based problems and work toward methods of coping. MIND, the mental health charity, also offers good advice. In one of its recent booklets (MIND, 1999. *Depression—Don't Let It Get You Down*. MIND and Pharmacy Healthcare; Mind Information, 15–19 Broadway, London E15 4BQ; Pharmacy Healthcare scheme, 1 Lambeth High Street, London SE1 7JN) about depression, it states that "pills are for symptoms, talking is for problems." You should also ensure that you eat a good nutritious diet (the brain needs proper nutrition) and avoid exposure to artificial pesticides, especially organophosphates (see Chapter 6), and excessive alcohol consumption. If you do have serious depression, however, it is important to seek medical help. Although modern antidepressants have side effects in some patients, it is better to take them than to suffer from serious depressive illness.

12. Cox, Peter, and Brusseau, Peggy, 1992. *Superliving: A Beginner's Guide to Medspeak*. Vermillion.

13. Boots the Chemist, 1998. *Breast Awareness—An Essential Guide: Be Enlightened, Not Frightened*. Published in association with the charity Breast Cancer Care.

14. *Sunday Correspondent*, 26 November 1989.

15. Alternative Therapy, British Medical Association, 1986.

16. Vickers, A., and Zollman, C., 1999. ABC of complementary medicine: acupuncture. *British Medical Journal*, 9 October, 973–6.

17. Gerson, M., 1958. *A Cancer Therapy: Results of Fifty Cases*. Gerson Institute, California; Forbes, Alec, 1984. *The Bristol Diet*. Century.

18. Greenwald, P., 1996. Chemoprevention of cancer. *Scientific Amercan*, Special Issue: What You Need to Know about Cancer, September, 96–100. See also the World Health Organization's International Agency for Research on Cancer website: http://who-pcc.iarc.fr/ the British National Formulary, 1998.
19. See, for example, section on cytotoxic (cell poisoning) drugs in the British National Formulary, 1998.

CHAPTER 2

1. Weinberg, Robert A., 1996. How cancer arises. *Scientific American*, Special Issue, What You Need to Know about Cancer, September, 62–70.
2. Pollack, M.N., and others, 1998. IGF-1 risk factor for prostate cancer. *Science*, 279, 563–6.
   Pollack, M.N.; Huynh, H.T.; and Lefebvre, S.P., 1992. Tamoxifen reduces serum insulin-like growth factor 1 (IGF-1). *British Cancer Research and Treatment*, 22, 91–100; Pollack, M.N., and others, 1988. Characterisation of insulin-like growth factor-1 (IGF-1) receptors of human breast cancer cells. *Biochemical Biophysical Research Communications*, 154(1), 326–31.
3. Oliff, Allen; Gibbs, Jackson B.; and McCormick, Frank, 1996. New molecular targets for cancer therapy. *Scientific American*, Special Issue, What You Need to Know about Cancer, September, 144–9.
4. Lichtenstein, P., and others, 2000. Environmental and heritable factors in the causation of cancer—analysis of cohorts of twins from Sweden, Denmark and Finland. *New England Journal of Medicine* 343(2), 78–85.
5. Davies, D.L., 2000. http://www.sfgate.com/cgi-bin/article.cgi?file=/chronicle/archive/2000/08/10/ED9161.DTL
6. Weinberg, Robert A., 1996. How cancer arises. *Scientific American*, Special Issue, What You Need to Know about Cancer, September, 62–70.
7. Jain, R.K., 1994. Barriers to drug delivery in solid tumours. *Scientific American*, July, 58–65.

CHAPTER 3

1. Trichopoulos, Dimitrios; Li, Frederick P.; and Hunter, David J., 1996. What causes cancer? *Scientific American*, Special Issue, What You Need to Know about Cancer, September, 80–5.
2. Ibid.
3. Boots the Chemist, 1998. *Breast Awareness—An Essential Guide:* Be Enlightened, Not Frightened. Published in association with the charity Breast Cancer Care.
4. Trichopoulos, Dimitrios; Li, Frederick P.; and Hunter, David J., 1996. What

causes cancer? *Scientific American*, Special Issue, What You Need to Know about Cancer, September, 80–5.

5. Holland, J.C., 1996. Cancer's psychological challenges. *Scientific American*, Special Issue, What You Need to Know about Cancer, September, 158–61.

6. http://www.who.int/nut/malnutrition_worldwide.htm

7. Parkin, D.M., and others, ed., 1997. *Cancer Incidence in Five Continents*. Vol 7. International Agency for Research on Cancer (WHO) Scientific Publications No. 143, Lyon. The data from the United States are from the Surveillance Epidemiology and End Results (SEER) Program of the National Cancer Institute.

8. http://who=pcc.iarc.fr/

9. Ibid.

10. Kliewer, E.V., and Smith, K.R., 1995. Breast cancer mortality among immigrants in Australia and Canada. *Journal of National Cancer Institute* 87(15), 1154–61. See also Cancer Research Campaign, 1996, Factsheet 6.2, Breast Cancer—UK.

11. Campbell, T.C., and Junshi, C., 1994. Diet and chronic degenerative disease perspectives from China. *American Journal of Clinical Nutrition* 59, Suppl., 11,535–615.

12. Rohan, T.E.; McMichael, A.J.; and Bagbursi, P.A., 1988. A population-based case control study of diet and breast cancer in Australia. *American Journal of Epidemiology* 128, 478–89; Howe, G.R., and others, 1990. Dietary factors and risk of breast cancer: combined analysis of 12 case-control studies. *Journal of the National Cancer Institute* 8, 561–9; Willet, Walter C., and others, 1987. Dietary fat and the risk of breast cancer. *New England Journal of Medicine*, 316, 22–28; Jones, D.Y., and others, 1987. Dietary fat and breast cancer in the National Health and Nutrition Examination Survey epidemiological follow-up study. *Journal of the National Cancer Institute* 79, 465–71.

13. Trichopoulos, Dimitrios; Li, Frederick P.; and Hunter, David J., 1996. What causes cancer? *Scientific American*, Special Issue, What You Need to Know about Cancer, September, 80–5.

14. Cramer, D.W., and others, 1989. Galactose consumption and metabolism in relation to the risk of ovarian cancer. *Lancet* 2, 66–71.

15. Stocks, P., 1970. Breast cancer anomalies. *British Journal of Cancer* 24, 633–43.

16. Maruchi, N., and others, 1977. Relation of food consumption to cancer mortality in Japan, with special reference to international figures. Gann, 68, 1–13.

CHAPTER 4

1. Cox, Peter, and Brusseau, Peggy, 1995. *LifePoints for Kids*. Bloomsbury.

2. Statistical Abstracts of the United States, 1994 edition.

3. Willett, W.C., and others, 1996. Strategies for minimizing cancer risk. *Sci-*

entific American, Special Issue, What You Need to Know about Cancer, September, 88–95.

4. Akre, James, ed., 1989. *Infant Feeding: The Physiological Basis*. WHO Bulletin, OMS Supplement, Vol. 67; Lawrence, Ruth A., 1994. *Breastfeeding: A Guide for the Medical Profession*. 4th ed. St. Louis: Mosby.

5. Lawrence, Ruth A., 1994. *Breastfeeding: A Guide for the Medical Profession*. 4th ed. St. Louis: Moseby.

6. Ibid.

7. Akre, James, ed., 1989. *Infant Feeding: The Physiological Basis*. WHO Bulletin, OMS Supplement, Vol. 67; Lawrence, Ruth A., 1994. *Breastfeeding: A Guide for the Medical Profession*. 4th ed. St. Louis: Mosby.

8. Ibid.

9. Ibid.

10. American Academy of Pediatrics Committee on Nutrition, 1992. The use of whole cows' milk in infancy. *Pediatrics* 89, 1105–9.

11. Anyon, C.P., and Clarkson, K.G., 1971. A cause of iron-deficiency anaemia in infants. *New Zealand Medical Journal* 74, 24–5.

12. Clyne, P.S., and Kulczycki, A., 1991. Human breast milk contains bovine IgG: relationship to infant colic? *Pediatrics* 87(4), 439–44; Wilson, J.F.; Lahey, M.E.; and Heiner, D.C., 1974. Studies on iron metabolism. V. Further observations on cow's milk-induced gastrointestinal bleeding in infants with iron-deficiency anemia. *Journal of Pediatrics*, 84, 335–44.

13. Pugh, R.H., 1981. Allergy to cows' milk protein. *Health Visitor* 54, 231–3.

14. Scott, F.W., 1990. Cow milk and insulin-dependent diabetes mellitus: is there a relationship? *American Journal of Clinical Nutrition* 51, 489–91.

15. Bahna, S.L., 1987. Milk allergy in infancy. *Annals of Allergy* 59, 131.

16. Dunea, G., 1982. Beyond the etheric. *British Medical Journal* 285, 428–9.

17. Kretchmer, N., 1981. The significance of lactose intolerance. In Paige, D.M., and Bayless, T.M., eds, *Lactose Digestion: Clinical and Nutritional Implications*. Baltimore: Johns Hopkins University Press.

18. Chiodini, R.J., and Hermon-Taylor, J., 1993. The thermal resistance of Mycobacterium paratuberculosis in raw milk under conditions simulating pasteurization. *Journal of Veterinary Diagnostic Investigation* 5, 629–31; Grant, I.R.; Ball, H.J.; and Rowe, M.T., 1996. Inactivation of Mycobacterium paratuberculosis in cows' milk at pasteurization temperatures. *Applied and Environmental Microbiology* 62, 631–6.

19. Institute of Food Science and Technology Position Statement, 1998. *Food Science and Technology Today* 12 (4), 223–8; http://www.ifst.org/hottop23.html

20. Ibid.

21. European Union Directive 70/524, February 1999.

22. U.S. Food and Drug Administration websites: http://vm.cfsan.fda.gov/~ear/m190-11.html; http://vm.cfsan.fda.gov/~ear/

23. Ingersoll, Bruce, 1990. Technology and Health: FDA Detects Drugs in Milk but Fails to Confirm Results. *Wall Street Journal*, 6 February, B6; Ingersoll, Bruce, 1990. Politics and Policy: GAO Says FDA Can't Substantiate Claims About Milk. *Wall Street Journal*, 21 November, A16; Ingersoll, Bruce, 1990. Technology & Health: FDA Plans a Nationwide Test of Milk for Antibiotics, Other Drug Residues. *Wall Street Journal*, 28 December, 10.

24. European Commission, Scientific Committee on Veterinary Measures Relating to Public Health, 1999. *Report on Public Health Aspects of the Use of Bovine Somatotropin*, 15–16 March.

25. Outwater, J.L., and others, 1997. Dairy products and breast cancer: the IGF-1, estrogen and bGH hypothesis. *Medical Hypotheses* 48, 453–61.

26. *Guardian*, 13 July 1999.

27. McCusker, R.H., 1998. Controlling insulin-like growth factor activity and the modulation of insulin-like growth factor binding protein and receptor binding. *Journal of Dairy Science*, 81, 1790–1800.

28. Institute of Food Science and Technology Position Statement. http://www.easynet.co.uk/ifst/hottop8a.htm

29. Eppard, P.J., and others, 1985. Effect of dose of bovine growth hormone on milk consumption: alpha-lactalbumin, fatty acids and mineral elements. *Journal of Dairy Science* 68(11), 3047–54. See also Cohick, W.S., and others, 1992. Regulation of insulin-like growth factor-binding proteins in serum and lymph of lactating cows by somatotropin. *Endocrinology* 130(3), 1508–14.

30. Mepham, T.B., and others, 1994. Safety of milk from cows treated with bovine somatotropin. *Lancet* 334, 19 November, 1445–6; Mepham, T.B., and Schonfield, P.N., 1995. *Health Aspects of BST Milk*, prepared for the International Dairy Federation Nutrition Week conference in Paris, France, June 1995.

31. Simpson and others, http://www.nal.usda.gov/ttic/tektran/glimpse/data/000007/75/0000077539.html

32. Miller, M.A., and others, 1989. Determination of insulin-like growth factor-1 (IGF-1) concentrations in raw pasteurized and heat treated milk. *Journal of Dairy Science* 72, Suppl. 1, 186–7.

33. Hankinson, Susan E., and others, 1998. Circulating concentrations of insulin-like growth factor-1 and risk of breast cancer. *Lancet* 351, 9 May, 1393–6.

34. Chan, J.M., and others, 1998. Plasma insulin-like growth factor-1 and prostate cancer risk: a prospective study. *Science* 279, 563–6.

35. Pollack, M.N.; Huynh, H.T.; and Lefebvre, S.P., 1992. Tamoxifen reduces serum insulin-like growth factor 1 (IGF-1). *British Cancer Research and Treatment* 22, 91–100.

36. Pollack, M.N., and others, 1998. IGF-1 risk factor for prostate cancer. *Science* 279, 563–6.

37. Chan, J.M., and others, 1998. Plasma insulin-like growth factor-1 and prostate cancer risk: a prospective study. *Science* 279, 563–6.

38. Holly, Jeff, 1998. Insulin-like growth factor-1 and new opportunities for cancer prevention. *Lancet* 351, 9 May, 1373–5.

39. Epstein, Samuel S., 1996. Unlabelled milk from cows treated with biosynthetic growth hormones: a case of regulatory abdication. *International Journal of Health Services* 26(1), 173–85.

40. Outwater, J.L.; Nicholson A.; and Barnard, N., 1997. Dairy products and breast cancer: the IGF-1, estrogen, and bGH hypothesis. *Medical Hypotheses* 48, 453–61.

41. Leonard, Rodney E., 1995. Codex at the crossroads: conflict on trade health. *Nutrition Week*, 25(26), 4–5. *Nutrition Week* is published by the Community Nutrition Institute, 910 17th Street, N.W., Suite 413, Washington, DC 20006.

42. European Commission. Health and Consumer Protection. Scientific Committee on Veterinary Measures Relating to Public Health—outcome of discussions. http://europa.eu.int/comm/dg24/health/sc/scv/out19_en.html

43. D'Ercole, J.A.; Underwood, L.E.; and Van Wyk, J.J., 1977. Serum somatomedin-C in hypopituaritism and in other disorders of growth. *Journal of Pediatrics* 90(3), 375–81. See also Cullen, K.J., and others, 1990. Insulin-like growth factor receptor expression and function in human breast cancer. *Cancer Research* 50, 48–53.

44. De Leon, D.D., and others, 1992. Effects of insulin-like growth factors (IGFs) and IGF receptor antibodies on the proliferation of human breast cancer cells. *Growth Factors* 6, 327–36.

45. Peyrat, J.P., and others, 1993. Plasma insulin-like growth factor 1 (IGF-1) concentrations in human breast cancer. *European Journal of Cancer* 29A(4) 492–7.

46. Ibid.

47. Musgrove, E.A., and Sutherland, R.I., 1993. Acute effects of growth factors on T471 breast cancer cell cycle progression. *European Journal of Cancer*, 29A(16), 2273–9.

48. Heldrin, C.N., and Westermark, B., 1984. Growth factors: mechanism of action and relation to oncogenes. *Cell* 37(9), 20.

49. Macaulay, V.M., 1992. Insulin-like growth factors and cancer. *British Journal of Cancer* 65, 311–20.

50. Underwood, L.E.; D'Ercole, J.A.; and Van Wyk, J.J., 1980. Somatomedin-C and the assessment of growth. *Pediatric Clinics of North America* 27(4), 771–82; Perdue, J.F., 1984. Chemistry, structure and function of insulin-like growth factors and their receptors: a review. *Canadian Journal of Biochemistry and Cell Biology* 62, 1237–45.

51. Outwater, J.L.; Nicholson, A.; and Barnard, N., 1997. Dairy products and breast cancer: the IGF-1, estrogen, and bGH hypothesis. *Medical Hypotheses* 48, 453–61.

52. European Commission. Health and Consumer Protection. Scientific Committee on Veterinary Measures Relating to Public Health—outcome of discussions. http://europa.eu.int/comm/dg24/health/sc/scv/out19_en.html

53. Council on Scientific Affairs, American Medical Association, 1991. Biotechnology and the American agricultural industry. *Journal of the American Medical Association* 265(11), 20 March, 1433.

54. Mepham, T.B., and Schonfield, P.N., 1995. Health aspects of BST milk, prepared' for the International Dairy Federation Nutrition Week conference in Paris, France, June 1995.

55. Challacombe, D.N., and Wheeler, E.E., 1994. Safety of milk from cows treated with bovine somatotropin. *Lancet* 344(17), 815.

56. Sell, C.; Rubin, R.; and Baserga, R., 1995. Insulin-like growth factor I (IGF-I) and the IGF-I receptor prevent etoposide-induced apoptosis. *Cancer Research* 55(2), 303–6.

57. Burton, Jeanne L., and others, 1994. A review of bovine growth hormone. *Canadian Journal of Animal Science* 74, 167–201.

58. Xian, C., 1995. Degradation of IGF-1 in the adult rat gastrointestinal tract is limited by a specific antiserum of the dietary protein casein. *Journal of Endocrinology* 146(2), 215; Thornburg, W., and others, 1984. Gastrointestinal absorption of epidermal growth factor in suckling rats. *American Journal of Physiology* 246, G80–5.

59. Outwater, J.L.; Nicholson, A.; and Barnard, N., 1997. Dairy products and breast cancer: the IGF-1, estrogen, and bGH hypothesis. *Medical Hypotheses* 48, 453–61.

60. Haraguchi, S., and others, 1992. Human prolactin regulates transfected MMTV LTR-directed gene expression in a human breast-carcinoma cell line through synergistic interaction with steroid hormones. *International Journal of Cancer* 52, 923–33.

61. Clevenger, C.V., and others, 1995. Expression of prolactin and prolactin receptor in human breast carcinoma: evidence for an autocrine/paracrine loop. *American Journal of Pathology* 146, 695–705.

62. Vonderhaar, B.K., 1989. Estrogens are not required for prolactin induced growth of MCF-7 human breast cancer cells. *Cancer Letters* 47, 105–10.

63. http://www.shef.ac.uk/uni/academic/a-c/csi/1997/pir2.html

64. Lochnan, H.A., and others, 1995. Functional activity of the human prolactin receptor and its ligands. *Molecular and Cellular Endocrinology* 114, 91–9.

65. http://mammary.nih.gov/reviews/tumorigenesis/Vonderhaar001/slides/introduction.html

66. Struman, I., and others, 1999. Opposing actions of intact and N-terminal fragments of the human prolactin/growth hormone family members on angiogenesis: an efficient mechanism for the regulation of angiogenesis. *Proceedings of the National Academy of Sciences of the United States of America* 96, 1246–51.

67. http://www.eurekalert.org/releases/upmc-bcc061699.html

68. Lawrence, Ruth A., 1994. *Breastfeeding: A Guide for the Medical Profession.* 4th ed. St. Louis: Mosby.

69. E.g., http://www.inter-medico.com/prolactn.html

70. Lawrence, Ruth A., 1994. *Breastfeeding: A Guide for the Medical Profession.* 4th ed. St. Louis: Mosby.

71. Poggi, S.H., and others, 1998. Using scanning electron microscopy to study mineral deposits in breast tissues. *American Mineralogist* 83, 1122–6.

72. Lee, J.R., 1996. *Natural Progesterone.* Oxfordshire: John Carpenter Publishing.

73. Wolford, S.T., and Argoudelis, C.J., 1979. Measurement of estrogens in cows' milk, human milk, and dairy products. *Journal of Dairy Science* 62(9), 1458–63.

74. Outwater, J.L.; Nicholson, A.; and Barnard, N., 1997. Dairy products and breast cancer; the IGF-1, estrogen, and bGH hypothesis. *Medical Hypotheses* 48, 453–61.

75. Royal society, 2000. Endocrine disrupting chemicals (EDCs). Document 06/00. Also available on www.roysoc.ac.uk

76. European Commission. Health and Consumer Protection. Scientific Committee on Veterinary Measures Relating to Public Health—outcome of discussions, 1999. http://europa.eu.int/comm/dg24/health/sc/scv/out19_cn.html

77. Allen, N.E., and others, 2000. Hormones and diet: low insulin-like growth factor-1 but normal bioavailable androgens in vegan man. *British Journal of Cancer* 83(1), 95–7.

78. Chan, J.M., and others, 1998. Plasma insulin-like growth factor-1 and prostate cancer risk: a prospective study. *Science* 279, 563–6.

79. Kradjian, R.M., 1994. *Save Yourself from Breast Cancer—Life Choices That Can Help You Reduce the Odds.* New York: Berkley Books.

80. "Milk Letter": http//www.afpafitness.com/milkdoc.htm

CHAPTER 5

1. Wright, K., 1996. A plea for prevention. *Scientific American,* Special Issue, What You Need to Know about Cancer, September, 99.

2. Report of Collaborative Group on Hormonal Factors in Breast Cancer, 1996. *Lancet* 347, 1713–27.

3. http://www.who.int/nut/malnutrition_worldwide.html

4. *The Times,* 2 November 1999.

5. Riggs, B.L., and others, 1987. Dietary calcium intake and rates of bone loss in women. *Journal of Clinical Investigation,* October, 80(4), 979–82.

6. Hegsted, D.M., 1986. Calcium and osteoporosis. *Journal of Nutrition* 116, 2316–9.

7. Kim, J.B., 1990. Fractured truths. *Bestways* 18(2), 26.

8. Ibid.

9. http://www.who.int/nut/malnutrition_worldwide.html

10. Dietary Reference Values for Food Energy and Nutrients for the United Kingdom. Department of Health, 1991.

11. Dietary Reference Values for Food Energy and Nutrients for the United Kingdom. Department of Health, 1991, p. 139, table 22.2.

12. Havala, S., and Dwyer, J., 1988. Position of the American Dietetic Association: vegetarian diets—technical support paper. *Journal of the American Dietetic Association*, 88(3), 352–5.

13. Barnard, N., 1993. *Food for Life*. New York: Crown Publishing.

14. Research Advances in Osteoporosis, 1990. Conference by the National Osteoporosis Foundation, the National Institutes of Health, and the American Society of Bone and Mineral Research, Arlington, Virginia, February.

15. Heaney, R.P., and Weaver, C.M., 1990. Calcium absorbability from kale. *American Journal of Clinical Nutrition* 51, 656–7.

16. Breslau, N.A., and others, 1988. Relationship of animal protein-rich diet to kidney stone formation and calcium metabolism. *Journal of Clinical Endocrinology and Metabolism* 66(1), 140–6.

17. Heaney, R.P., and Recker, R.R., 1982. Effects of nitrogen, phosphorus, and caffeine on calcium balance in women. *Journal of Laboratory and Clinical Medicine* 99(1), 46–55.

18. Hopkins, P.N., and others, 1995. Higher plasma homocysteine and increased susceptibility to adverse effects of low folate in early familial coronary artery disease. *Arterosclerosis, Thrombosis, and Vascular Biology* 15(9), 1314–20; Robinson and others, 1995. Hyperhomocysteinemia and low pyridoxal phosphate; common and independent reversible risk factors for coronary artery disease. *Circulation* 92(10), 2825–30; Aro, G.A., and Key, K.F., 1997. Plasma homocysteine and cardiovascular disease mortality. *Lancet* 349, 397.

19. Pritchard, K.I., and others, 1996. Increased thromboembolic complications with concurrent tamoxifen and chemotherapy in a randomized trial of adjuvant therapy for women with breast cancer. *Journal of Clinical Oncology* 14(10), 2731–8.

20. Gooderham, M.J., and others, 1996. A soy protein isolate rich in genistein and daidzein and its effects on plasma isoflavone concentrations, platelet aggegation, blood lipids and fatty acid composition of plasma phospholipid in normal men. *Journal of Nutrition* 126, 2000–6.

21. Greenwald, Peter, 1996. Chemoprevention of cancer. *Scientific American*, Special Issue, What You Need to Know about Cancer, September, 96–9.

22. Kurzer, M.S., and Xu, X., 1999. Dietary phytoestrogens. *Annual Reviews of Nutrition* 17, 353–81.

23. Shurtleff, William, and Aoyagi, Akiko, 1975. *The Book of Tofu*. Autumn Press.

24. Kurzer, M.S., and Xu, X., 1999. Dietary phytoestrogens. *Annual Reviews of Nutrition* 17, 353–81. See also Jenkins, D.J., and others, 2000. Effect of soy protein foods on low-density lipoprotein oxidation and ex vivo sex hormone receptor activity—a controlled crossover trial. *Metabolism* 49(4), 537–43.

25. U.K. Ministry of Agriculture, Fisheries and Food, advice as reported in the *Sunday* (London) *Times*, 1999.

26. Willet, W.C., 1994. Micronutrients and cancer risk. *American Journal of Clinical Nutrition* 59, Suppl., 1162S–5S. See also Willett, Walter C.; Colditz, Graham A.; and Mueller, Nancy A., 1996. Strategies for minimizing cancer

risk. *Scientific American*, Special Issue, What You Need to Know about Cancer, September, 88–95.

27. Greenwald, Peter, 1996. Chemoprevention of cancer. *Scientific American*, Special Issue, What You Need to Know about Cancer, September, 96–9.

28. Levy, J., and others, 1995. Lycopene is more potent inhibitor of human cancer cell proliferation than either A-carotene or B-carotene. *Nutrition and Cancer* 24, 257–66.

29. Nagasawa, H., and others, 1995. Effects of lycopene on spontaneous mammary tumour development in SHN virgin mice. *Anticancer Research* 15, 1173–8.

30. Willett, Walter C.; Colditz, Graham A.; and Mueller, Nancy A., 1996. Strategies for minimizing cancer risk. *Scientific American*, Special Issue, What You Need to Know about Cancer, September, 88–95.

31. Ortega, R.M., and others, 1996. Functional and psychic deterioration in elderly people may be aggravated by folate deficiency. *Journal of Nutrition* 126, 1992–9.

32. Hopkins, P.N., and others, 1995. Higher plasma homocysteine and increased susceptibility to adverse effects of low folate in early familial coronary heart disease. *Arterosclerosis, Thrombosis, and Vascular Biology* 15(9), 1314–20.

33. Jenkins, D.J., and others, 2000. Effect of soy protein foods on low-density lipoprotein oxidation and ex vivo sex hormone receptor activity—a controlled crossover trial. *Metabolism* 49(4), 537–43.

34. Adlercreutz, H., 1998. Phytoestrogens: State of the Art. In Baush-Goldbohm, S.; Kardinaal, A.; and Serra, F., eds., Third Workshop, Doorweth, Netherlands, 17–18 April, European Commission.

35. Phipps, W.R., and others, 1993. Effect of flax seed ingestion on the menstrual cycle. *Journal of Clinical Endocrinology and Metabolism* 77(5), 1215–9.

36. www.flax.com.fda

37. Greenwald, Peter, 1996. Chemoprevention of cancer. *Scientific American*, Special Issue, What You Need to Know about Cancer, September, 96–9.

38. Coghlan, Andy, 1999. Crunch time for cancer. *New Scientist* 164 (2212), 13 November.

39. Pinto, J.T., and others, 1999. Effects of garlic thioallylic derivatives on growth, glutathione concentration, and polyamine formation of human prostate carcinoma cells in culture. *American Journal of Clinical Nutrition*. See also Li, G., and others, 1995. Antiproliferative effects of garlic constituents in cultured human breast cancer cells. *Oncology Reports* 2, 787–91.

40. http://www.3mistral.co.uk/garlic/cancer.htm See also http://www.mskcc.org/rande/pharmacology/189.html

41. Greenwald, Peter, 1996. Chemoprevention of cancer. *Scientific American*, Special Issue, What You Need to Know about Cancer, September, 96–9.

42. Doll, R., and Peto, R., 1981. *The Causes of Cancer: Quantitative Estimates of Avoidable Risks of Cancer in the United States Today*. New York: Oxford University Press.

43. Lang, T., and Clutterbuck, C., 1991. *P Is for Pesticides*. Ebury Press, Random Century Group.

44. McMichael, A.J., 1993. *Planetary Overload—Global Environmental Change and the Health of the Species*. Cambridge: Cambridge University Press.

45. Lang, T., and Clutterbuck, C., 1991. *P Is for Pesticides*. Ebury Press, Random Century Group.

46. http://www.radian.com/standards and http://ro-systemsnet/atrazine.html

47. Stevens and others, 1994. http://www-oem.ucdavis.edu~beaumont/Agrichem/ herbicides/triazine/triazine.html See also Stevens, J.T., and Sumner, D.D., 1991. Herbicides. In *Handbook of Pesticide Toxicology*, vol. 3, *Classes of Pesticides*. Toronto: Academic Press, 1317–1408; *Environmental Endocrine Disrupters: A Handbook of Property Data*, 1999.

48. http://who-pcc.iarc.fr/

49. Hambridge, K.M.; Casey, C.E.; and Krebs, N.F., 1986. Zinc. In Mertz, W., ed., *Trace Elements in Human and Animal Nutrition*, 5th ed. London: Academic Press.

50. McCusker, R.H., 1998. Controlling insulin-like growth factor activity and the modulation of insulin-like growth factor binding protein and receptor binding. *Journal of Dairy Science* 81, 1790–1800.

51. Simpson and others. Effect of exogenous estradiol on plasma concentrations of somatotropin, insulin-like growth factor 1, insulin-like growth factor–binding protein activity, and metabolites in ovariectomised Angus and Brahman cows. http://www.nal.usda.gov/ttic/tektran/glimpse/data/000007/75 /0000077539.html

52. The Toronto *Globe and Mail*, 31 July 1999.

53. Vikse, R., and others, 1999. Heterocyclic amines in cooked meat. *Tidsskr Nor Laegeforen* 119(1), 45–9.

54. Skog, K., and others, 1997. Polar and non-polar heterocyclic amines in cooked fish and meat products and their corresponding pan residues. *Food Chemical Toxicology* 35(6), 555–65.

55. Hendler, S.S., 1990. *The Doctors' Vitamin and Mineral Encyclopedia*. New York: Simon and Schuster.

56. Hetzel, B.S., and Maberly, G.F., 1986. Iodine. In Mertz, W., ed., *Trace Elements in Human and Animal Nutrition*, 5th ed. London: Academic Press.

57. Eskin, B.A., and others, 1976. Rat mammary gland atypia produced by iodine blockade with perchlorate. *Cancer Research* 35(9), 2332–9. See also Eskin, B.A., 1978. In Schrauzer, G.N., ed., *Inorganic and Nutritional Aspects of Cancer*, New York: Plenum Press, 293–304. This reference is quoted in Crouse, and others, 1983. Geochemistry and Man: Health and Disease 1. Essential Elements. In Thornton, I., ed., *Applied Environmental Geochemistry*, London: Academic Press, 267–308.

58. Johnson, C., 1999. Environmental controls in iodine deficiency disorders (IDD). *Earthworks*, 9 November, 3.

59. Simopoulos, A.P., 1991. Omega-3 fatty acids in health and disease and in growth and development. *American Journal of Clinical Nutrition* 54, 438–63.

60. Simopoulos, A.P., 1991. Omega-3 fatty acids in health and disease and in

growth and development. *Amercan Journal of Clinical Nutrition* 54, 438–63. See also Fernandes, G., and Venkatraman, J.T., 1993. Role of omega-3 fatty acids in health and disease. *Nutrition Research* 13, S19–S45.

61. Reported in the London *Evening Standard*, 17 March 1989. See also Willet, W.C., 1994. Micronutrients and cancer risk. *American Journal of Clinical Nutrition* 59, Suppl., 1162S–5S.

62. Hunter, David J., and Willett, Walter C., 1993. Diet and body build: diet, body size and breast cancer. *Epidemiologic Reviews* 15(1), 110–32.

63. Ingram, A.J., and others, 1995. Effects of a flaxseed and flax oil diet in a rat—⅚ renal ablation model. *American Journal of Kidney Disease*, 25(2), 320–9.

64. Obermeyer, W.R., and others, 1995. Chemical studies of phytoestrogens and related compounds in dietary supplements—flax and chaparral. *Proceedings of the Society for Experimental Biology and Medicine*. See also Obermeyer, W.R., and others, 1993. Flaxseed lignans, isolation metabolism, and biological effects. *Federation of American Societies for Experimental Biology Journal* A863.

65. Dupont, J., and others, 1989. Food safety and health effects of canola oil. *Journal of the American College of Nutrition* 8, 360–75.

66. Kohlmeier, L., and others, 1997. Adipose tissue trans fatty acids and breast cancer in the European Community Multicenter Study on Antioxidants, Myocardial Infarction, and Breast Cancer. *Cancer Epidemiology, Biomarkers and Prevention* 6(9), 705–10.

67. Koletzko, B., 1992. Trans fatty acids may impair biosynthesis of long-chain polyunsaturates and growth in man. *Acta Paediatrica*, 81, 302–6.

68. Fasano, A., and Horvath, K., 2000. University of Maryland Center for Celiac Research, Multi-Center Serological Screening Study Results. May 20 (Link); Horvath, K., and others, 1996. First epidemiological study of gluten intolerance in the United States. *Gastroenterology*, April.

69. Halsted, C.H., 1996. The many faces of celiac disease. *New England Journal of Medicine*, 334, 18; Goggins, and others, 1994. Celiac disease and other nutrient related injuries to the gastrointestinal tract. *American Journal of Gastroenterology* 89(8), S2–S13.

70. Forbes, Alec, 1984. *The Bristol Diet*. London: Century.

71. Ingram, A.J., and others, 1995. Effects of flaxseed and flax oil diets in a rat—⅚ renal ablation model. *American Journal of Kidney Disease* 25(2), 320–9.

72. Lee, S., and others, 1999. Monitoring of drinking water in terms of natural organic matter and disinfection by-products. Proceedings of the 2nd International Symposium on Advanced Environmental Monitoring, Kwangju, Korea.

73. Herrick, D., 1996. Cryptosporidium and Giardia: should you be concerned? *Water Well Journal* 50(4), 49, 44–6.

74. Jankun, Jerzy, and others, 1997. Why drinking green tea could prevent cancer. *Nature*, 15 June, 561. See also Greenwald, Peter, 1996. Chemoprevention

of cancer. *Scientific American*, Special Issue, What You Need to Know about Cancer, September, 96–9.

75. Jankun, Jerzy, and others, 1997. Why drinking green tea could prevent cancer. *Nature*, 15 June, 561.

76. Campion, K., 1986. *Vegetarian Encyclopaedia*, London: Century Hutchinson.

77. Jankun, Jerzy, and others, 1997. Why drinking green tea could prevent cancer. *Nature*, 15 June, 561.

78. http://research.kib.ki.se/e-uven/public/51419.html

79. Lockwood, K., and others, 1994. Apparent partial remission of breast cancer in "high risk" patients supplemented with nutritional antioxidants, essential fatty acids and coenzyme Q_{10}. *Molecular Aspects of Medicine* 15, Suppl, 231–40; Lockwood, K.; Moesgaard, S.; and Folkers, K., 1994. Partial and complete regression of breast cancer in patients in relation to dosage of coenzyme Q_{10}. *Biochemical and Biophysical Research Communications* 199(3), 1504–8; Lockwood, K., and others, 1995. Progress on therapy of breast cancer with vitamin Q_{10} and the regression of metastases. *Biochemical and Biophysical Research Communications* 212(1), 172–7.

CHAPTER 6

1. Cited in *Better Nutrition*, November 1989, 14(2).

2. Levander, O.A., 1986. Selenium. In Mertz, W., ed., *Trace Elements in Human and Animal Nutrition*. 5th ed. London: Academic Press.

3. Spallholz, J.E., and Stewart, J.R., 1989. Advances in the role of minerals in immunobiology. *Biological Trace Element Research* 19(3), 129–51.

4. Levander, O.A., 1986. Selenium. In Mertz, W., ed., *Trace Elements in Human and Animal Nutrition*. 5th ed. London: Academic Press.

5. Shamberger, R.J.; Tytko, S.A.; and Willis, C.E., 1976. *Archives of Environmental Health* 31, 231.

6. Knekt, Paul, and others, 1988. Selenium deficiency and increased risk of lung cancer. Abstract of paper read at the 4th International Symposium on Selenium in Biology and Medicine, Tubingen, West Germany, July.

7. Reinhold, U., and others, 1988. Selenium deficiency and lethal skin cancer. Abstract of paper read at the 4th International Symposium on Selenium in Biology and Medicine, Tubingen, West Germany, July.

8. Lockwood, K., and others, 1994. Apparent partial remission of breast cancer in "high risk" patients supplemented with nutritional antioxidants, essential fatty acids and coenzyme Q_{10}. *Molecular Aspects of Medicine* 15, Suppl, 231–40. See also Lockwood, K.; Moesgaard, S.; and Folkers, K., 1994. Partial and complete regression of breast cancer in patients in relation to dosage of coenzyme Q_{10}. *Biochemical and Biophysical Research Communications* 199(3), 1504–8; Lockwood, K., and others, 1995. Progress on therapy of breast cancer

with vitamin Q_{10} and the regression of metastases. *Biochemical and Biophysical Research Communications* 212(1), 172–7.

9. Monographs on the Evaluation of the Carcinogenic Risk of Chemicals to Man, 1982. Geneva: World Health Organization, International Agency for Research on Cancer, 1972–present. Vol. 29, p. 282; see also Osihi, Shinshi, 1990. Effects of phthalic acid esters on testicular mitochondrial functions in the rat. *Archives of Toxicology* 64(2), 143–5.

10. Holland, J.C., 1996. Cancer's psychological challenges. *Scientific American*, Special Issue, What You Need to Know about Cancer, September, 158–61.

11. Heason, P., *Deep Relaxation*. Tape available from 37 Tollerton Lane, Tollerton, Nottingham, U.K.

12. Based on Holland, J.C., 1996. Cancer's psychological challenges. *Scientific American*, Special Issue, What You Need to Know about Cancer, September, 158–61.

13. Trichopoulos, Dimitrios; Li, Frederick P.; and Hunter, David J., 1996. What causes cancer? *Scientific American*, Special Issue, What You Need to Know about Cancer, September, 80–5.

14. Levy, Len, 1998, Biomed II: Exposure to low-level benzene, In Institute for Environment and Health, Annual Report, p. 76.

15. Pearson, J.K., 2000. *The Air Quality Challenge*, American Society of Automotive Engineers and HMSO.

16. North Atlantic Treaty Organization, 1988. International Toxicity Equivalency Factor (I-TEF) method of risk assessment for complex mixtures of dioxins and related compounds: pilot study on international information exchange on dioxins and related compounds. CCMS Report No. 176. Washington, D.C.: Environmental Protection Agency; Department of Health, 1995. Statement by the Committee on Toxicity of Chemicals in Food, Consumer Products and the Environment on the U.S. EPA draft health assessment document for 2,3,7,8-tetrachlorodibenzo-*p*-dioxin (TCDD) and related compounds. London: Department of Health.

17. EPA Dioxin Reassessment Summary, 1994. Vol. 1. CERI/ORD Publication Center, U.S. Environmental Protection Agency, April.

18. MAFF, 1997. Dioxins and PCBs in retail cows' milk in England. *Food Surveillance Information Sheet*, No. 136, December. London: Ministry of Agriculture, Fisheries and Food.

19. Tanabe, S., 1988. PCB problems in the future: foresight from current knowledge. *Environmental Pollution* 50, 5–28.

20. Department of the Environment, 1989. Dioxins in the environment. *Pollution Paper*, No. 27. London: HMSO.

21. MAFF, 1997. Dioxins and polychlorinated biphenyls in fish oil dietary supplements and licensed medicines. *Food Surveillance Information Sheet*, No. 106. London: Ministry of Agriculture, Fisheries and Food.

22. MAFF, 1996. Dioxins in human milk. *Food Surveillance Information Sheet*, No. 88. London: Ministry of Agriculture, Fisheries and Food.

23. MAFF, 1996. Polychlorinated biphenyls in food—UK Dietary Intakes. *Food Surveillance Information Sheet,* No. 89. London: Ministry of Agriculture, Fisheries and Food.

24. Keith, L.H., and Johnson, T., eds, 1997. *Environmental Endocrine Disruptors: A Handbook of Property Data.* New York: John Wiley and Sons.

25. Shin, K.J., and others, 1999. Development of a bioassay system for identification of endocrine disrupters. Proceedings of the 2nd International Symposium on Advanced Environmental Monitoring, Kwangju, Korea.

26. Soto, A.M., and others, 1992. An in culture bioassay to assess the estrogenicity of xenobiotics. In Colborn, T.C., ed., *Chemically-Induced Alterations in Sexual and Functional Development: The Wildlife/Human Connection,* Vol. 21. Princeton Scientific Publishing, 295–309. See also Soto, A.M., and others, 1995. The E-SCREEN assay as a tool to identify estrogens: an update on estrogenic environmental pollutants. In *Estrogens in the Environment: Environmental Health Perspectives,* 113–22.

27. Davis, D.L., and others, 1997. Environmental influences on breast cancer risk. *Science and Medicine,* May/June.

28. Colborn, T.; Dumanoski, D.; and Myers, J.P., 1996. *Our Stolen Futures.* New York: Dutton, Penguin Books.

29. Dyson, T., 1999. Prospects for feeding the world. *British Medical Journal* 319, 988–91.

30. Reuters, 8 October 1998.

31. McMurry, Laura M.; Oethinger, Margaret; and Levy, Stuart B., 1998. Triclosan targets lipid synthesis. *Nature* 394 (6693), 531–2.

32. Trichopoulos, Dimitrios; Li, Frederick P.; and Hunter, David J, 1996. What causes cancer? *Scientific American,* Special Issue, What You Need to Know about Cancer, September, 80–5.

CHAPTER 7

1. Campbell, T.C., and Junshi, C., 1994. Diet and chronic degenerative disease perspectives from China. *American Journal of Clinical Nutrition* 59, Suppl., 11,535–615.

2. Peto, R., and others, 2000. Smoking, smoking cessation, and lung cancer in the UK since 1950: combination of national statistics with two case-control studies. *British Medical Journal* 321, 323–9.

3. Bok, D., 1990. In *Universities and the Future of America.* Durham, N.C.: Duke University Press.

4. Glantz, S.A., 1996. *Times Higher Education Supplement,* 6 September, 15, and Glantz, S.A., and others, 1996. *The Cigarette Papers.* Berkeley: University of California Press.

5. Kradjian, R.M., 1994. *Save Yourself from Breast Cancer—Life Choices That Can Help You Reduce the Odds.* New York: Berkley Books.

6. Packham, D.E., 1999. Impacts of commercialisation and privatisation on capabilities for scientific advice: oracles or scapegoats? (U.K.) Institution of Professional Managers and Specialists Conference notes, October. See also Packham, David, and Tasker, Mary, 1997. Industry and the academy—a Faustian contract. *Industry and Higher Education*, April, 85–90.

7. Ibid.

8. Jasanoff, S., 1997. Civilization and madness: the great BSE scare of 1996. *Public Understanding of Science* 6, 221–32.

9. McMichael, A.J., and Powles, J.W., 1999. Human numbers, environment, sustainability and health. *British Medical Journal* 319(9), 977–80.

Further Reading

❧

Blauer, Stephen, 1989. *The Juicing Book*. New York: Avery Publishing Group.

Bremness, Lesley, 1990. *World of Herbs*. London: Ebury Press.

Conil, Christopher and Jean, 1993. *New Tofu Recipes*. W. Foulsham and Co.

Daniel, R., 2000. *Living with Cancer*. London: Robinson.

Jaffrey, Madhur, 1981. *Eastern Vegetarian Cooking*. London: Arrow Books.

Lamont, Heather, 1988. *The Gourmet Vegan*. London: Victor Gollancz.

Pert, C.B., 1997. *Molecules of Emotion: Why You Feel The Way You Feel*. London: Simon and Schuster.

Ramsay, Ray, 1994. *Easy Thai Cooking*. Wellingborough: J. B. Fairfax Press.

Shurtleff, William, and Aoyagi, Akiko, 1988. *The Book of Tofu: Food for Mankind*. Berkeley, Calif.: Ten Speed Press.

Sen, J., 1996. *Healing Foods Cookbook*. London: Thorsons.

So Yan-Kit, 1992. *Classic Food of China*, London: Macmillan.

Thorson Editorial Board, 1989. *The Complete Raw Juice Therapy*. London: Thorsons, HarperCollins.

Wheater, Caroline, 1993. *Juicing for Health*. London: Thorsons, HarperCollins.

Index